PREVENTION'S
System of Health and Natural Healing

Healing Yourself with Food

By the Editors of **PREVENTION** *Magazine*
Health Books

Edited by Edward Claflin

Rodale Press, Inc.
Emmaus, Pennsylvania

Library of Congress Cataloging-in-Publication Data

  Healing yourself with food / by the editors of Prevention Magazine Health Books : edited
    by Edward Claflin.
        p.   cm. —(Prevention's system of health and natural healing)
    Includes index.
    ISBN 0-87596-242-4 hardcover
    1. Nutrition. 2. Diet therapy. I. Claflin, Edward. II. Prevention Magazine Health Books.
  III. Series.
  RA784.H39 1995
  615.8'54—dc20   94–42424

Distributed in the book trade by St. Martin's Press

2   4   6   8   10   9   7   5   3   1   hardcover

OUR MISSION

We publish books that empower people's lives.

RODALE ❦ BOOKS

Information about Daily Values of Nutrients: Throughout this book, we usually refer to Daily Values (DV) when we're discussing the recommended amounts of vitamins or minerals in your daily diet. The DV for each nutrient is a reference number that's found in the listing of "Nutrition Facts" on food labels. The list shows what percentage of nutrients—compared to the recommended daily amount—you get in each serving of that particular food. Each DV is expressed as a percentage of the current nutrition recommendations (set by the government) based on a daily diet of 2,000 or 2,500 calories, and the serving size is based on what most people actually eat. But your own nutrient needs may be higher or lower, depending on your daily calorie intake.

While nutrition and ingredient information is mandatory, food companies are required to list only two vitamins (A and C) and two minerals (calcium and iron). Many companies, however, voluntarily list other nutrients on their labels.

Though the DVs usually apply to both men and women, recommendations sometimes differ for each sex. In those cases, we refer to Recommended Dietary Allowances (RDA) rather than Daily Values.

Prevention's System of Health and Natural Healing
Healing Yourself with Food Editorial and Design Staff

Managing Editor: Edward Claflin
Senior Editor: Matthew Hoffman
Food Editor: Jean Rogers
Writers: Brian Chichester, Sid Kirchheimer, Peggy Morgan, Laura Wallace-Smith, Mark Wisniewski
Art Director and Series Designer: Debra Sfetsios
Cover Designer: Debra Sfetsios
Senior Designers: Helene Wald Berinsky, Joseph Perez
Designers: Christopher R. Neyen, Timothy M. Teahan
Photo Editor: Susan Pollack
Copy Editor: Jane Sherman
Head Researchers: Carlotta Cuerdon, Bernadette Sukley
Research Associates: Christine Dreisbach, Theresa Fogarty, Carol J. Gilmore, Sandra Salera Lloyd, Christina Orchard-Hays, Sally A. Reith, John Waldron
Nutritionist: Anita Hirsch
Permissions: Anita Small
Production Coordinator: Jodi Schaffer
Office Staff: Roberta Mulliner, Julie Kehs, Bernadette Sauerwine

Prevention Magazine Health Books
Editor-in-Chief, Rodale Books: Bill Gottlieb
Executive Editor: Debora A. Tkac
Art Director: Jane Colby Knutila
Research Manager: Ann Gossy Yermish
Copy Manager: Lisa D. Andruscavage

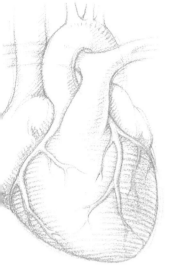

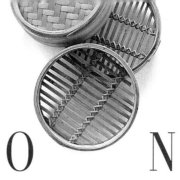

C O N T

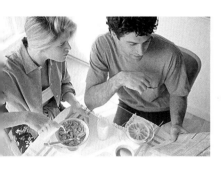

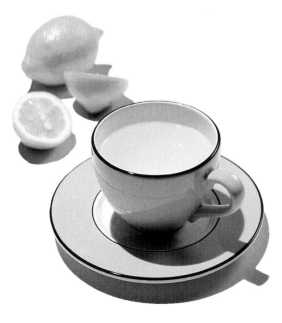

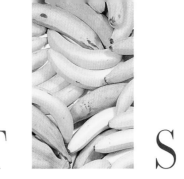

E N T S

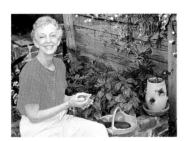

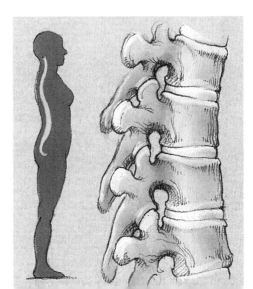

Introduction

THE PRACTICAL SCIENCE OF NUTRITIONAL HEALING

I had an epiphany the other day—you know, one of those sudden revelations that clarifies everything about a topic or issue.

I was walking down the aisle of a local supermarket and there, next to the other cereals—next to a box filled with green marshmallows and a cereal that could have been manufactured by Godiva instead of General Mills—was a box full of . . . rice bran. Rice bran?

Now, this wasn't a cereal manufactured by Health Heaven or Purer Than Thou—some small company specializing in so-called health foods. This was a product from one of America's leading manufacturers of cereals, and they had decided to sell . . . rice bran.

And right then and there, I knew—I knew that food and nutrition in America were never going to be the same.

This product is a result of what I like to call The Practical Science of Nutritional Healing. This science—the same science that helped create all of the advice in *Healing Yourself with Food*—doesn't just tell us that good foods are good for you, or even that fiber is good for you. Everybody knows that. It tells you exactly which foods are good for exactly which conditions—just the same way that a doctor prescribes a specific drug for a specific disease. It says that there isn't just one kind of bran (like oat bran). There's also corn bran, wheat bran and rice bran (of course) and each of these can prevent or heal disease in a very specific way.

The editors at *Prevention* Magazine Health Books have taken every detail of The Practical Science of Nutritional Healing—they've read thousands of scientific studies and interviewed hundreds of doctors and researchers—and distilled it into one book: *Healing Yourself with Food*. Now, when you're at the supermarket, you'll know why rice bran is good for you—and you'll also know the four best nuts to lower cholesterol . . . the best type of bean to prevent colon cancer . . . the best poultry for boosting your immune system . . . and hundreds of other practical tips. In fact, you'll have an epiphany, too—a revelation that you can be as healthy as you want to be, just by choosing the right foods.

See you in Aisle 7.

Yours for better health,

Bill Gottlieb

Bill Gottlieb
Editor-in-Chief, *Prevention* Magazine Health Books

PART ONE

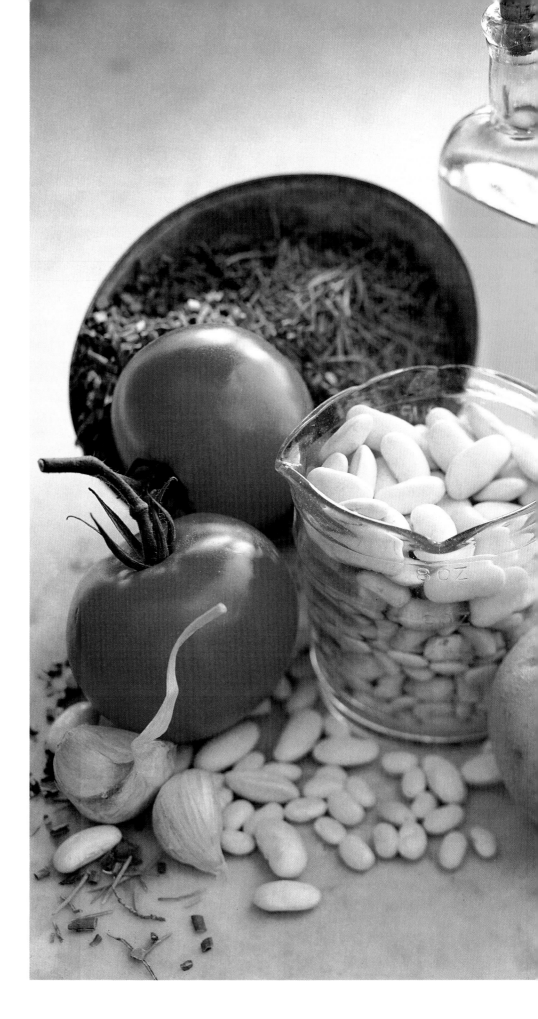

Fat-Fighting Diets to Scrub Your Arteries Clean

Choose

the foods

that

roll back

your risks

Y ou've got a lot going for you. A miraculous heart that thumps away with remarkable predictability. Highways and byways of blood vessels that transport nutrients to all your hungry cells. And a system of energy transfer that's highly efficient.

A body system like this deserves respect. And that's exactly what you're giving it when you exercise regularly, eat high-nutrition, low-fat foods and keep disaster-makers like cigarettes out of reach.

Knowing this, you probably have a good idea of what it takes to keep your cholesterol down, avoid high blood pressure and prevent heart attack and stroke. But knowing what to do, and doing something about it, are two different things. When it comes to looking after your heart and arteries, you can significantly reduce your risk just by choosing the food you eat, no matter what your age, sex or family history of heart disease.

That's why you'll find scores of tips, tactics, guidelines, recipes and menus in the next three chapters. All are part of a practical system for eating well—a system that will help you fight heart disease, America's number-one health risk.

We've combed the research, talked to leading experts and interviewed numerous doctors to find out what will work for you. And as you'll discover in the following pages, the news is good.

Quick Tips to Clobber Cholesterol

N ow that "beef" and "eggs" have become the newest breed of four-letter words, you may find your nerves standing on end whenever someone mentions the latest-learned evils about cholesterol.

Well, it's because of cholesterol that your nerves can do that. Despite a reputation for breaking more hearts than Don Juan, cholesterol isn't all bad. In fact, your body needs it—and produces up to 2,000 milligrams in the liver each day—to build every cell and nerve sheath in your body. Cholesterol also helps produce sex hormones like estrogen and testosterone and bile acids to digest food and transform the sun's rays into vitamin D inside your body for strong bones and teeth. Without cholesterol, we couldn't live.

But with too much of it, we can die. The 500,000 deaths by heart attack and the three million strokes that occur in the United States every year are usually the result of excess cholesterol swimming through our blood vessels. It accumulates along artery walls, where it hardens and eventually narrows blood vessels, choking off the supply of blood—a condition known as atherosclerosis, or hardening of the arteries.

Since the body manufactures all the cholesterol it needs, this excess generally comes from only one source: "For the vast majority of Americans, high cholesterol is the result of their diet,"

FROM YOUR FOOD TO YOUR BLOOD

Half of all Americans have high cholesterol because of the way they eat. Dietary cholesterol is found only in "animal" food sources such as meat and dairy products. It's not in "plant" food sources such as fruits, vegetables or beans, so eating more of these foods can help you reach the American Heart Association's recommendation of less than 300 milligrams of cholesterol a day. That's the cholesterol equivalent of 1⅓ egg yolks.

The table below shows desirable, borderline and undesirable levels of cholesterol, measured three ways. Total cholesterol is the amount of cholesterol in your blood. A reading of under 200 is desirable; anything over 240 is considered dangerous. HDL cholesterol is high-density lipoproteins—the "good" cholesterol that scours artery walls. LDL cholesterol is low-density lipoproteins, the "bad" cholesterol. You can lower LDLs by eating more soluble fiber and other heart-healthy foods.

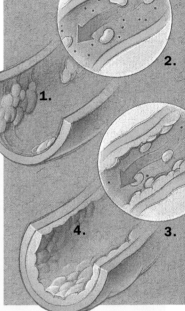

In a normal, healthy artery (1), the HDL cholesterol helps to clear out LDL (2). Even though some arterial plaque builds up on the blood vessel walls, it isn't a health risk. If your blood has too many LDLs and not enough HDLs, the LDLs create a buildup of plaque on the artery walls (3), which can cause blockage (4).

Test	Your Level (mg/dl)		
	Desirable	Borderline	Undesirable
Total cholesterol	Below 200	200–240	Above 240
HDL cholesterol	Above 45	35–45	Below 35
LDL cholesterol	Below 130	130–160	Above 160

says John LaRosa, M.D., dean of research at George Washington University School of Medicine in Washington, D.C., and past president of the American Heart Association's (AHA) Nutrition Committee. Cholesterol is found in varying amounts in all animal products (animals also need it to live). It is abundant in such all-American staples as meat, eggs and whole-milk dairy foods.

"There is a definite link between a diet high in cholesterol and an increased risk of coronary heart disease—even independent of other known risk factors like smoking or not getting enough exercise," adds epidemiologist Richard B. Shekelle, Ph.D., of the University of Texas Health Science Center in Houston, who headed the first significant long-term study on dietary cholesterol in the United States. (His study on 2,107 men, which began in 1957, paved the way for much of what we know about diet and cholesterol.) "And the more cholesterol you eat, the higher the risk," he says.

IT BEGAN WHEN THE RABBITS DIED

Until a few decades ago, this mild-mannered crystalline steroid alcohol did its handiwork with little fanfare in our blood, bile, nerve fibers, organs and adrenal glands. Few people knew—or cared—what cholesterol was.

But that started to change in 1911, when a Russian researcher, Dr. Nikolai Anitschkov, did an experiment—the first of hundreds that would eventually put cholesterol on everyone's "Least Wanted List." He discovered that when he fed rabbits a diet of egg yolk, a high amount of cholesterol from the yolk entered their bloodstream, as food does in order to fuel our bodies. The cholesterol formed crusty deposits called plaques along artery walls, which narrowed blood vessels as though they were clogged pipes. The rabbits died.

Since then, there have been hundreds of other studies that basically prove the same thing: The more cholesterol in your blood, the more you're

CLAMS HELP SINK LIPOS

One of the biggest fish stories to ever come from the briny deep is the whopper that all shellfish are swimming in cholesterol.

Granted, shrimp and some other types of "surf" can clog your arteries—especially when deep-fried or drowning in butter. But researchers tout a few treasures from Davy Jones's locker: namely, clams, oysters, crabs and mussels.

Studies at the University of Washington found that if you go for these nautical nibbles instead of the meat, eggs and cheese consumed by the typical American, you can help lower a type of cholesterol called very-low-density lipoprotein. In these studies, researchers found that this type of cholesterol plummeted by one-half after only three weeks on a diet that included these types of seafood. In the same studies, beneficial HDLs actually rose.

About 20 small steamed clams have only 60 milligrams of cholesterol—what you'd find in three syrup-topped pancakes. Clams also pack plenty of nutritional punch—and they're easy to prepare.

To remove sand from clams, add a handful of cornmeal and some salt to a bowl of water, add the live clams and let soak for an hour (*1*). Use a stiff vegetable brush to clean the shells (*2*). Place the clams in a pot, add two inches of water and cover. Bring to a boil and steam for five to ten minutes (*3*). When the shells open, the clams are ready (*4*). If they don't open, the clams are inedible.

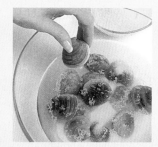

1. Soak.

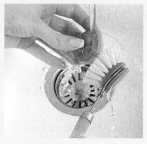

2. Scrub.

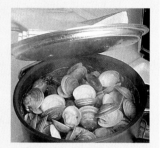

3. Steam.

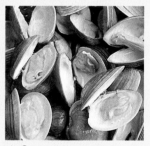

4. Serve.

tempting fate. For every 1 percent increase in your blood cholesterol level, researchers have learned, your risk of heart disease increases by 2 percent. The good news is that for every percentage point you lower your cholesterol, your heart disease risk is cut by twice that amount.

"The problem is, there aren't many

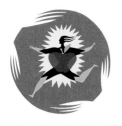

BREAKTHROUGHS IN HEALING

foods that actually lower your cholesterol," says Margo Denke, M.D., a noted heart disease researcher and assistant professor of medicine at the University of Texas Southwestern Medical School in Dallas, who is a member of the AHA's Nutrition Committee. "But it's clear that there are many foods that can raise your cholesterol level." And they include some that you'd never suspect.

DON'T HAVE A BEEF ONLY WITH BEEF

Pity Old MacDonald. Once he was praised in song for his collection of critters that helped feed a nation. But now we're singing the blues over the beef, milk and eggs that have come from his much-ballyhooed farm. And why not? These farm-fresh foods are loaded with cholesterol.

So we've taken to eating more poultry and marine life, thinking we're doing our arteries a favor. We're also consuming 3½ billion fewer eggs each year than in 1970, thinking that by passing on the morning omelet, we're in the clear—cholesterol-wise. Yet half of all Americans still have cholesterol levels over the "desirable" range of 200 milligrams per deciliter (mg/dl). And many are well over the "dangerous" level of 240 mg/dl.

What gives?

"The idea that any single food causes cholesterol problems, or will be enough to control them, is just plain silly," says George Washington University's Dr. LaRosa. "I have patients who give up eating eggs for breakfast and wonder why their cholesterol is still high. And unfortunately, they're not alone in that thinking."

While it's a good idea to limit your diet of beef, eggs and other foods that you know are high in cholesterol, keep in mind that cholesterol is in all animal foods to some degree. Even the so-called healthy choices offer their own cholesterol traps. Here's some advice.

Avoid all organ meats. In animals (as in humans), the highest concentrations of cholesterol are found in organs such as the liver, brain and gonads. And since beef has more cholesterol than other meats, people assume that red meat organs such as calves' liver are the worst. *Trap:* Turkey and chicken liver have even more cholesterol than beef liver. In fact, a single serving of beef liver has less than two-thirds the cholesterol of turkey and chicken liver. And roe, the eggs of fish, has more cholesterol than any cut of red meat.

Look to shellfish. Many cholesterol-conscious people consider shellfish strictly taboo—mostly because they know that shrimp is loaded with cholesterol. But other forms of shellfish are extremely healthful: Clams, oysters and mussels are lower in cholesterol and fat than even chicken and pack a lot more nutrition per bite.

Keep an eye out for eggs. Bite for bite, egg yolks have more cholesterol than any other food in the American diet. Just 1⅓ yolks give us more cholesterol than the AHA recommends we eat in an entire day. *Trap:* Many of the 233 eggs consumed each year by the typical American come from baked goods and from other "prepared" foods—not from the morning omelet. That's why it's essential to read food labels to find out whether eggs are included in the packaged or prepared foods you're eating.

Eat more often, not more. Some people assume that the less they eat, the less cholesterol they consume—so they skip meals like breakfast and lunch. *Trap:* Your body needs food, so eating a big meal to make up for several skipped ones can trigger a large release of insulin, which in turn causes the liver to produce more cholesterol. *Better:* To prevent this surge of cholesterol, nibble throughout the day—ideally, a "nibble" every hour or so.

THE REAL PROBLEM: OUR DIET IS SATURATED WITH FAT

But the biggest cholesterol trap is the belief that blood cholesterol rises only

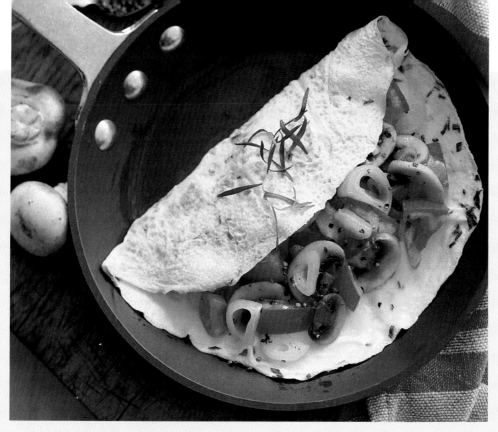

A breakfast favorite with a low-cholesterol profile, this mushroom-onion omelet is made with fat-free egg substitute.

Chop the Cholesterol from Egg-y Favorites

You don't have to steer clear of eggs just because you're watching your cholesterol. You can have as many as you like, as long as you use fat-free egg substitute—or watch your yolk consumption.

The Zero-Cholesterol Mushroom-Onion Special

1	cup thinly sliced mushrooms
1	cup thinly sliced onions
1½	cups fat-free egg substitute
2	tablespoons water
1	teaspoon Dijon mustard
1	tablespoon minced fresh tarragon or parsley
½	teaspoon ground black pepper
2	teaspoons margarine

Place the mushrooms and onions in a 4-cup glass measure and cover loosely with plastic wrap. Microwave on high for 3 minutes, or until the vegetables are softened. Drain off any liquid.

In a medium bowl, whisk together the egg substitute, water, mustard, tarragon or parsley and pepper.

In a large no-stick frying pan over medium heat, melt the margarine and swirl the pan to coat the bottom. Pour in the egg mixture. As the egg begins to set, pull the outer edges toward the center with a fork or spatula; allow uncooked portions to run underneath. Continue until just set.

Sprinkle with the mushrooms and onions. Fold the omelet in half. Cut into 2 sections and transfer to serving plates.

Makes 2 servings.

Note: If you don't have a microwave, place the mushrooms and onions in a large no-stick frying pan. Add 1 tablespoon water and cook, covered, over medium heat until the vegetables are softened and the mushrooms release their juices. Remove the lid and cook until the liquid evaporates.

Per serving: 139 calories, 2.7 g. fat (18% of calories), 2 g. dietary fiber, 0 mg. cholesterol, 311 mg. sodium.

when you eat foods high in dietary cholesterol.

"Actually, it's entirely possible to eat a totally cholesterol-free diet and still raise your blood cholesterol level," says Dr. LaRosa, one of the nation's foremost researchers on heart disease. "In fact, people do it all the time."

All you have to do is eat a lot of saturated fats. And unfortunately, that's something we have no problem doing: The all-American diet is fatty enough, with more than one-third of our total calories coming from fat—sometimes as much as one-half.

It's not as though we've cornered the market on high-fat eating. People in Greece, Italy and other nations around the Mediterranean Sea actually consume almost as much fat as Americans, yet they have a surprisingly low rate of heart disease. The reason: Their fat is "healthier"—it's mostly monounsaturated and polyunsaturated fats from plant-based foods.

But we tend to eat up to four times as much animal-based saturated fats as those Europeans. "Many people focus on limiting their dietary cholesterol, so they think if a label says 'No Cholesterol,' they're in the clear," says Dr. LaRosa. "But in fact, saturated fat is anywhere from three to five times as powerful as dietary cholesterol itself in raising your blood cholesterol."

So while it's important to limit dietary cholesterol to 300 milligrams a day (compared to the 450 milligrams most Americans consume), it's even more important to be on the lookout for saturated fats.

Lighten up. A cup of whole milk has about 9 grams more fat than skim—over 5 of them saturated. A serving of regular yogurt has nearly 5 more grams of saturated fat than nonfat yogurt. Even so-called healthy foods can be as high in fat as they are in nutrients. But if you switch to low-fat or nonfat versions of these and other foods, you can easily cut up to 20 grams or more of saturated fat each day—and you won't

lose out on the vitamins and minerals.

In fact, the light versions are often more nutritious: Nonfat yogurt, for instance, has *more* calcium, riboflavin, magnesium, potassium, zinc and vitamin B_{12} than its higher-fat counterparts—and it contains an enzyme that helps lower cholesterol.

Consider new condiments. Butter has only 11 milligrams of cholesterol per teaspoon but gets all of its calories from fat. Some salad dressings that are "cholesterol-free" can contain 10 grams of fat per tablespoon! Mayonnaise is nearly all fat, with 11 grams per tablespoon. Keep in mind that most Americans use these toppings very liberally, which is why they can add as much as 30 grams of fat a day without even knowing they're doing it.

Instead of these high-fat flavorings, use fat-free butter substitutes, nonfat dressings, fat-free yogurt and other healthy alternatives. Better yet, develop a yen for mustard, ketchup, horseradish, chili sauce, relish and salsa. Besides adding zest to meals, they're all very low in fat and have no cholesterol.

Veg out. Most foods that are high in cholesterol are also high in saturated fats, so they do a double-whammy on your arteries, says Richard Milani, M.D., director of the Cardiovascular Health Center at the Oschner Clinic in New Orleans. "Animal fats are among the worst," he says.

A great way to slash saturated fats is to make vegetables the focal point of your meals. Shoot for at least one vegetarian meal a day, and have no more than one three-ounce serving a day of lean meat, fish or poultry—in other words, a serving that's about the size of a deck of cards. Red meat should be consumed no more than twice or three times a week.

READING BETWEEN THE LIES

The single best thing you can do to reduce saturated fats is open your eyes—and read between the lies . . . er, *lines*, of food labels. Here's how.

NIBBLE AWAY AT CHOLESTEROL

It's not just *what* you eat that can determine your cholesterol level—it's also *when* you eat it. Large meals cause the release of high levels of insulin, which stimulates the liver's production of cholesterol.

By eating the same amount of calories in smaller, more frequent meals, you can control cholesterol by keeping insulin "more steady," says Thomas Wolever, M.D., Ph.D., associate professor of nutritional sciences at the University of Toronto.

"In our studies, people experienced a significant drop in total cholesterol after a couple of weeks when they had smaller meals spread out throughout the day—basically nibbling every hour or so—instead of three bigger meals. But the key isn't the number of meals you eat; it's spreading out your calories so you eat approximately the same amount at each sitting."

Just to make sure it could be done, we divided a typical day's menu into nine separate meals. Here's the result—a total of 2,276 calories, with less than 20 percent coming from fat.

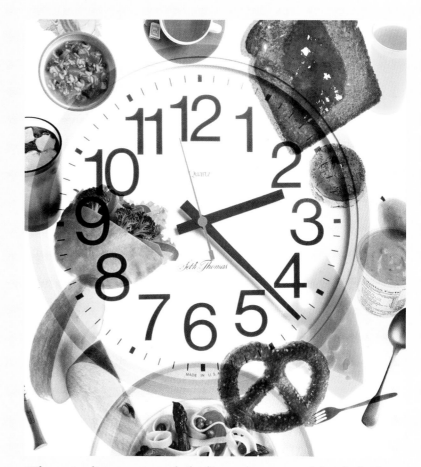

When you divvy up your daily diet and eat around the clock, the result is lower cholesterol, doctors say.

EARLY MORNING

2 slices wheat toast
2 teaspoons jam
1 sliced apple
1 cup brewed tea
Total calories: 255

BREAKFAST

¾ cup orange juice
1 cup oatmeal
¼ cup skim milk
1 glass water
Total calories: 229

MIDMORNING SNACK

1 bagel
¼ cup skim ricotta cheese
¼ teaspoon cinnamon
1 cup herbal tea
Total calories: 252

LUNCH

1 cup turkey vegetable soup
1 small tossed green salad
2 tablespoons low-calorie Italian
    dressing
1 slice Italian bread
1 teaspoon olive oil
2 glasses water
Total calories: 292

MIDAFTERNOON SNACK

1 cup low-fat fruit yogurt
1 pear
1 glass water
Total calories: 329

LATE-AFTERNOON SNACK

1 large pretzel
1 ounce Lite Jarlsberg cheese
Total calories: 140

DINNER

11 ounces frozen pasta primavera
1 apple
2 glasses water
Total calories: 361

MIDEVENING SNACK

Sliced raw vegetables (1 carrot,
    1 cup broccoli, ½ pepper)
⅓ cup yogurt cheese dip
1 pita bread pocket
1 glass water
Total calories: 248

LATE-EVENING SNACK

3 cups air-popped popcorn
1 tablespoon sunflower seeds
1 tablespoon almonds
1 cup herbal tea
Total calories: 170

Do your math. The AHA recommends that no more than one-third of your fat intake—which means only 10 percent of total calories—should come from saturated fats. To figure that 10 percent amount, all you have to do is check food labels for the Daily Value (DV). Keep your total daily intake below 100 percent of the DV for saturated fats, and you've met your goal.

The DVs are based upon a daily diet of 2,000 calories and a recommendation of no more than 65 grams of total fat and 20 grams of saturated fats per day. If your calorie intake is lower or higher, the grams of fat can be less or more. Women who consume 1,600 calories a day, for instance, should stay below 53 total grams of fat—or 18 grams of saturated fats. Men who average 2,500 calories daily should shoot for a total of less than 80 fat grams, or 25 grams of saturated fats.

Check the serving size. Packages that are labeled "single-serve" often contain two "suggested" servings—yet fat content is calculated on a per-serving basis. So be sure to read the suggested serving size before you eat, or you may get double the amount of fat that you calculated.

Be hip to hydrogenation. Take notice of the word "hydrogenated" on food labels. Hydrogenation is a process in which hydrogen is added to cheaper (and heart-healthier) unsaturated fats to give them the texture and taste of more expensive animal fats. *Trap*: People assume that because vegetable oils are considered heart-healthy, they're in the clear. In reality, hydrogenated vegetable oils have, in effect, become partially saturated in a way that will raise your cholesterol levels just as much as animal fats.

Stick to no-stick pans. Butter contains more than two grams of saturated fat per mere teaspoon (and few folks coat their frying pans with only one teaspoon). Many cooking oils are no better—containing 120 calories per tablespoon and getting 100 percent of

those calories from fat. "One of the best ways to cut down the amount of fat in your diet is to use as little cooking oil as possible—or even better, use no-stick pans," says Robert Nicolosi, Ph.D., professor of clinical science and director of cardiovascular research at the University of Massachusetts in Lowell and chairman of the AHA's Nutrition Committee.

If you don't use no-stick pans for cooking, use no-stick spray oil products, such as PAM. Because you use so little, spray oil is lower in fat and calories than butter and other oils, and contains no cholesterol.

Don't fall for the "No Cholesterol" line. From peanut butter to crackers, you'll notice that scores of products proudly boast that they contain no cholesterol. They shouldn't! Remember, cholesterol comes only from animal sources—and most prepackaged foods don't include these spoilable ingredients. Instead, pay attention to the fat content: Many of these "no cholesterol" products will still raise your cholesterol.

FIBER: AN OUNCE OF PREVENTION

Until now, you've heard about what you shouldn't eat in order to lower your cholesterol. Well, there is one type of food that you should eat for the same result—and the more you consume, the better.

"Dietary fiber fills you up, so you eat less food. And that's good for many people, since obesity is also a risk factor

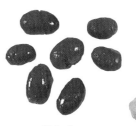

Baked beans ▼

Chick-peas ▶

GET KEENO ON BEANO

Beans, beans, good for the heart . . . hey, you know the rest.

But now there's a product that helps to control bean-induced gas: Beano, which is sold over the counter at drugstores and supermarkets, contains an enzyme that helps the body break down indigestible sugars in beans while they're still in the stomach.

Just splash a few drops on your first forkful of beans. It's safe and effective, but people who have diabetes or are allergic to mold or penicillin shouldn't use Beano without first checking with their doctor.

Butter beans ▶

Black beans ▶

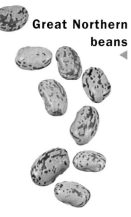

Great Northern beans

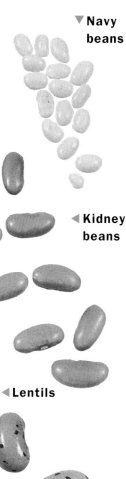

▼ Navy beans

◄ Kidney beans

◄ Lentils

◄ Pinto beans

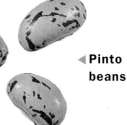

◄ Cranberry beans

Chock-Full of Beans

Beans are a great source of soluble fiber, which helps lower cholesterol. But some are better than others. The list below gives fiber amounts for ½ cup of some popular types of beans.

- *Kidney beans: 2.8 g.*
- *Cranberry beans: 2.7 g.*
- *Butter beans: 2.7 g.*
- *Baked beans, canned: 2.6 g.*
- *Black beans: 2.4 g.*
- *Navy beans: 2.2 g.*
- *Lentils: 2.0 g.*
- *Pinto beans: 1.9 g.*
- *Great Northern beans: 1.4 g.*
- *Chick-peas: 1.3 g.*

Mixed-Bean Soup

As long as you have beans in the pantry—never mind what kind—you have the makings of a heart-healthy soup that you can heat up and serve any time. Here's one that only gets better when you add more varieties of flavorful beans to the stockpot.

1½	cups mixed dried beans, soaked overnight
3	cups defatted chicken stock
3	cups water
1	cup diced onions
1	cup diced carrots
1	cup frozen corn
1	cup diced celery
1	clove garlic, minced
1	teaspoon dried thyme
½	teaspoon dried oregano
½	teaspoon ground black pepper
	Pinch of ground red pepper
2	tablespoons balsamic or red wine vinegar

Drain the beans and place in a 4-quart pot. Add enough cold water to cover the beans by about 2". Bring to a boil over high heat, reduce the heat to medium and cook for 1 hour. Drain. Return the beans to the pot.

Add the stock, water, onions, carrots, corn, celery, garlic, thyme, oregano, black pepper and red pepper. Bring to a boil over high heat, then reduce the heat

to medium. Partially cover the pan and simmer for 1 hour, or until the beans are very tender. If desired, use a potato masher to crush some of the beans to help thicken the soup. Stir in the vinegar.

Makes 6 servings.

Note: You may use any combination of beans. Some markets sell ready-made mixtures of five or more beans, or you can make your own blend by using up small quantities of beans that you have on the shelf. Chick-peas take longer to cook than other varieties, so you might want to forgo them in favor of navy beans, red or pink kidney beans, black beans, mung beans, adzuki beans, pinto beans, baby lima beans, cranberry beans or cannellini beans. You can also add small quantities of red, green or brown lentils and some yellow or green split peas, which cook quickly and help thicken the soup.

Per serving: 194 calories, 1.3 g. fat (6% of calories), 9.2 g. dietary fiber, 0 mg. cholesterol, 83 mg. sodium.

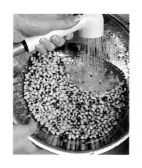

COOKING WITHOUT GAS

Unfortunately, dried beans will never totally run out of their own special brand of octane, but there's a way you can prepare them to cut back on the gas-producing substances. First, rinse the beans thoroughly under running water as shown. Pour boiling water over the rinsed beans to completely cover them. Allow the beans to soak for at least four hours, then remove any beans that have floated to the top. Drain the rest and cook them in fresh water.

for heart disease," says dietitian Rosemary Newman, R.D., Ph.D., professor of foods and nutrition at Montana State University in Bozeman, who has studied fiber and its relationship to cholesterol since the early 1980s. Besides filling you up, high-fiber foods tend to be very low in calories and fat, so they're really great for any weight-loss plan.

"But even more important, fiber can actually help lower cholesterol by preventing the absorption of fats and cholesterol," adds Dr. Newman.

It doesn't take much. One to three ounces a day of oat bran, oatmeal or other high-fiber food has been found to lower cholesterol levels an average of 5 to 10 percent. You can achieve even better results with more fiber—but it has to be the right kind.

There are two kinds of fiber, and while both are important to health, only one has proven to be effective in lowering cholesterol. It's called soluble fiber. It's abundant in beans, in fruit and in grains like oats, barley and rye. Soluble fiber gets its name because it dissolves in water to form a gel. This process, Dr. Newman and other researchers believe, helps lower cholesterol.

"The theory is that since it's soluble, it forms a gel-like material that keeps the cholesterol and fat molecules from getting to the interior wall of the intestines, where they are absorbed," she says. "And when these materials aren't absorbed, they are excreted through bowel movements."

Ever since the first finding in 1979 that soluble fiber could be part of a cholesterol-lowering regimen, various studies—including those by Dr. Newman and her colleagues—have documented the heart-helping effectiveness of soluble fiber.

The other type of dietary fiber, insoluble fiber, is found in vegetables, cereals and grains like wheat. Insoluble fiber is important to our overall diet, but since it doesn't "gel" in the

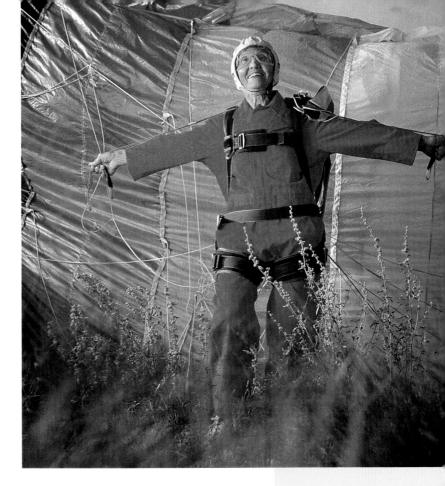

body, it's not as effective at keeping fats and cholesterol from being absorbed. "It offers some benefit by increasing bulk and speeding the progress of material through the intestines," Dr. Newman adds.

Most Americans don't get enough of either type of fiber. But here's how to get your fill of soluble fiber to help lower cholesterol.

Don't follow the 25/25 rule. According to the AHA, we should eat at least 25 grams of total dietary fiber a day. (In reality, women only eat 11 grams a day, while men have 18.)

Of that 25 grams, most experts recommend that 25 percent should come from soluble sources—about 6½ grams worth. "That's fine if you don't have a cholesterol problem, but if you're eating fiber to lower cholesterol, you should eat up to double that amount—so half of your fiber comes from soluble sources," says Dr. Newman. "That translates to over 12 grams a day for the average person."

Make cereal a snack. In just five minutes, you could be on the road to a

Because of a lifetime of good dietary habits, Corena Leslie still enjoys an active lifestyle at age 92—including skydiving to celebrate her 90th birthday. "I definitely make sure that every meal I eat is low in fat and high in fiber," says the resident of Peoria, Arizona.

IT'S NEVER TOO LATE TO LOWER

Changing bad eating habits can do you a lot of good—and it's never too late to start. "It doesn't take long to see some improvement—just a few weeks," says Dr. Rosemary Newman of Montana State University.

She knows of what she speaks: After studying the effects of fiber on cholesterol for more than a decade, she says people average a 15 percent reduction in cholesterol levels after just three weeks on a diet high in soluble fiber—no matter what their age. That decrease translates to a 30 percent drop in risk of heart attack. "My own cholesterol dropped 25 points in three weeks after I started adding about three ½-cup servings of rolled oats a day," says Dr. Newman.

diet that's much higher in fiber. "Perhaps the easiest way to get a five-gram booster is with cereals, since there are so many high-fiber choices," says George L. Blackburn, M.D., Ph.D., associate professor of surgery at Harvard Medical School and chief of the Nutrition/Metabolism Laboratory with the Cancer Research Institute at New England Deaconess Hospital in Boston. All it takes is a ⅓- to ½-cup serving of a cold, high-fiber cereal (or a cup of cooked hot cereal).

Hot or cold, bran cereals are quick and easy to fix. So, whether or not you have cereal for breakfast, fix a bowl of bran cereal for a good, filling snack anytime during the day.

Consume more legumes. For even more fiber, add beans to your diet whenever you can. By adding ½ cup of cooked kidney beans to salads, you'll add nearly seven grams of fiber, and nearly three grams of that is soluble. Or pour on ½ cup of cooked pinto beans for more than three grams of total fiber and about two grams of soluble fiber.

Go bonkers over barley. Oat bran may get the fame—and with good reason, since it's an excellent source of soluble fiber. But research shows that barley may be just as effective at lowering cholesterol. Studies at Texas A&M University in College Station show that adding a mere three grams of milled brewer's grain (which comes from barley) to the diet each day reduced LDL cholesterol an average of 6.5 percent after one month. Those having the same amount of barley oil saw drops of 9.5 percent.

Neither milled brewer's grain nor barley oil—which were used in the study—is available at food stores. You can get whole-grain barley flour at most health food stores, however, and it's a good substitute for regular wheat flour. So the next time you're baking, replace some of the wheat flour with whole-grain barley flour. Since the barley variety is higher in soluble fiber, a little goes a long way. (Barley has no gluten,

which is a necessary ingredient in some recipes, so you may not be able to make a 100 percent substitution.)

Take your multivitamins. While the best-known drawback of fiber—gas—is quite apparent (at least to those around you), there is one other potential problem: Large amounts of fiber sometimes interfere with your body's absorption of iron, zinc and other nutrients from food, especially if you do not have a balanced diet. But you can get a boost by taking a daily multivitamin. Just read the label to make sure it contains iron and zinc as well as a full complement of vitamins.

Fiber up before you pig out. Dr. Newman believes when you eat fiber may be as significant as what you eat when it comes to reducing cholesterol levels. "Instead of just eating oatmeal for breakfast and getting it out of the way, my belief is that you should have most of your fiber with your fattiest meal of the day in order to have it work most effectively. So if you're having a steak, have beans at that meal—or maybe 30 minutes before. Since soluble fiber inhibits the absorption of dietary fats, it makes sense that it would be most effective when we're having the most of those dietary fats."

A SOLUBLE-FIBER BOOSTER

If you find that it's difficult to boost soluble fiber with foods alone, you can get some help from psyllium (pronounced *silly-um*).

Created from the ground-up seed husks of a plant grown in India, psyllium is usually taken as a powder mixed with water and juice. For years, people have used this concentrated form of soluble fiber as a bulk-forming laxative. But research has shown that adding psyllium to a diet that's already low in fat can further reduce both total and LDL cholesterol, according to Dennis Sprecher, M.D., a cardiologist and director of the Lipid Research Clinic at the University of Cincinnati.

In one study, Dr. Sprecher found re-

FIBER-UP WITH A SUMMER SALAD

Eating a high-fiber diet isn't always a picnic—but there's a tasty way to get heaps of fiber in one salad. Pick high-pectin fruits and you'll be well on your way to lowering cholesterol.

Although best known as the gel in jellies and jams, pectin may be as effective as oat bran in lowering cholesterol. It blocks absorption of fats and dietary cholesterol and keeps them from entering the bloodstream, says noted researcher Dr. James Cerda of the University of Florida College of Medicine, whose pectin studies are famous among the cholesterol-watching medical community.

Fruits such as apples, grapefruit, oranges and bananas (as well as vegetables like carrots and beets) are among the top sources of this soluble fiber. (See the values at right for the amount of pectin in each three-ounce serving.)

According to Dr. Cerda, pectin-rich foods have other health-giving benefits. Among them:

◼ Many of the fruits and vegetables highest in pectin are also rich in antioxidant vitamins, shown to protect against heart disease (as well as other diseases).

◼ Pectin-rich foods suppress the appetite. And the less you eat, the less cholesterol and fat you consume.

◼ Some research shows that pectin seems to inhibit the formation of atherosclerosis, or "hardening of the arteries," the disease caused by high cholesterol.

▲ **Pineapple**
(<0.1 gram of pectin)

Apple ▶
(0.7 gram of pectin)

▲ **Peach**
(0.6 gram of pectin)

▲ **Bananas**
(0.4 gram of pectin)

▲ **Pear**
(0.7 gram of pectin)

▲ **Grapefruit**
(0.7 gram of pectin)

Grapes ▶
(0.3 gram of pectin)

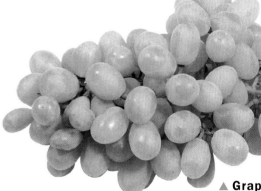

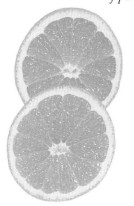

▼ Orange
(0.9 gram of pectin)

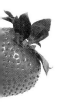

◄ Strawberries
(0.5 gram of pectin)

▼ Watermelon
(0.1 gram of pectin)

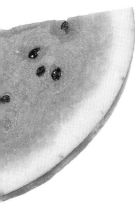

◄ Plum
(0.5 gram of pectin)

ductions in total cholesterol of more than 4 percent and decreases in LDL levels of more than 6 percent when study participants added ten grams of psyllium per day to a low-fat diet.

Just be sure to check with your doctor before using psyllium, Dr. Sprecher advises, because it can alter the absorption of medications you may be using. Also, you need to be sure to drink lots of water if you're taking a soluble supplement like psyllium.

THE FACTS ON FLAX

Raw flaxseed doesn't seem like the kind of fibrous food you'd like to have in a sandwich. But studies show this seed could be a powerful natural cholesterol controller.

In a study by the Jordon Research Group in Montclair, New Jersey, researchers found that when people began eating six slices of flax loaf daily instead of six slices of regular bread, their average total cholesterol fell about 10 percent, while the more harmul LDL cholesterol went from an average of 162 mg/dl down to 133. Beneficial HDL cholesterol did not go down at all. The big drop in total cholesterol translates into a probable reduction in heart attack risk of some 30 to 40 percent.

To make flax loaf, use a blender or coffee mill to grind the seeds to the consistency of cornmeal. Then substitute flaxseed meal for a portion of the cornmeal or flour in a regular bread recipe. As a general rule, ⅓ cup of flaxseed yields 1 cup of meal.

But start slowly—flaxseed is high in fiber, which can cause gassiness and bloating if you are not used to it. Another reason to ease into eating flaxseed bread is the possibility of an allergic reaction. Start with a small piece of bread, about the size of a penny, the first day. If you have any problems, see a doctor before eating more.

PECTIN: PRODUCTIVE PRODUCE

You don't have to eat like a Kentucky Derby favorite to get the fiber you need. And even better, you don't have to pass gas like one, either.

A type of fiber called pectin that's found in fruits and vegetables can lower cholesterol in the same way as oat bran: It helps prevent dietary cholesterol and fat from entering the bloodstream. "But pectin also seems to affect the enzymes in the liver that produce cholesterol. The more pectin you eat, the less cholesterol is produced by the liver," says professor of medicine and leading pectin researcher James Cerda, M.D., director of the Nutrition Research Laboratory at the University of Florida College of Medicine in Gainesville.

While no one's suggesting that you completely abandon bran, here's how to get more soluble fiber in your diet from pectin.

Grab a grapefruit. It's one of the highest sources of pectin available, with nearly 0.7 gram per three-ounce serving. That's significant, because in Dr. Cerda's studies, people with high cholesterol due to a poor diet and exercise habits had an average 12 percent reduction when eating the amount of pectin found in one to two grapefruit. "And they got those results by simply adding grapefruit to their diet; they made no other changes in their diet or lifestyle and did nothing else to help lower their cholesterol," he says. Other fruits that are rich in pectin include oranges, bananas, apples, strawberries, peaches, pears, plums and grapes.

Harvest some high-pectin veggies. Pectin is also abundant in vegetables such as lettuce, spinach, soybeans, carrots, beets, brussels sprouts, cabbage, potatoes, onions and peas, adds Dr. Cerda. So every time you add these vegetables to a salad or serve them with a meal, you're doing your arteries a favor.

Spread it out. "Since no meal goes by without having fat, it's best to divide your pectin into even doses throughout the day," says Dr. Cerda. "It's better to have three-quarters of a grapefruit for breakfast, lunch and dinner than to eat two grapefruit in one sitting."

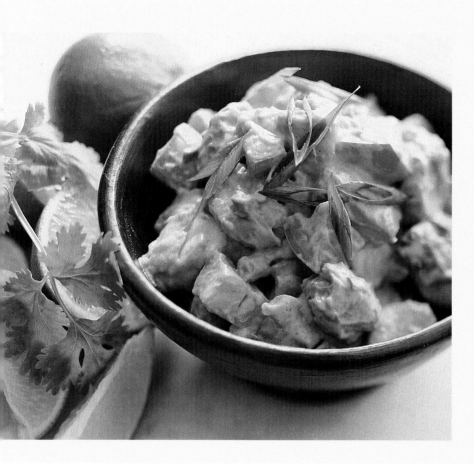

Good-Fat Avocado

You might not expect to find a secret weapon against cholesterol in a guacamole dip. After all, its main ingredient—avocado—has long been taboo among dieters, and with good reason: A single avocado has about 300 calories and nearly 30 grams of fat, half of the daily recommended amount for someone on a 1,800-calorie diet.

But an Australian study showed that a high-fat, avocado-rich diet can have a real impact on cholesterol levels. Two groups of women were placed on low-fat diets. The first group's dietary fat was then boosted 10 to 15 percent with the addition of ½ to 1½ avocados a day. Despite the high fat content of the avocado-rich diet, the women in the group that had the avocado-rich diet ended up with lower total cholesterol readings.

Reason: The fat in avocado is mostly monounsaturated—the kind that lowers LDLs but not HDLs.

FAT WITH EFFECT: THE MONOS HAVE IT

Not all fat is bad. In fact, as with cholesterol, you'd die without it. Fat stores our body's energy, and it's needed to build healthy hair and skin and to help regulate body temperature. Fat also insulates nerves with a protective covering. And the fat surrounding vital internal organs like the heart and kidneys helps to protect them from jolts and blows.

So any time we talk about losing fat for the sake of a healthy heart, we mean losing the fat we don't want—the kind that clogs arteries and contributes to heart disease and overweight.

But dietary fat—the oily blobs found in so many foods—comes in different forms. To get plenty of fat for nutrition and protection and still do your heart a favor, you need to be selective about the kind of fat you get in your food.

You already know about the "wrong" type—saturated fats that raise blood cholesterol. But you can actually lower blood cholesterol if you consume plenty of the "right" fats—namely monounsaturated and polyunsaturated fats. Unlike saturated fat, which is concentrated in meats and many dairy products, the unsaturated varieties are found in plant sources like fruits, vegetables, legumes and certain cooking oils, most notably olive oil.

Monounsaturates and polyunsaturates seem to work differently inside the body than saturated fats, according to Dr. Milani of the Oschner Clinic in New Orleans. "While a diet that's high in saturated fats tends to produce more cholesterol in the blood, polys and monos seem to have the opposite effect. They seem to produce less cholesterol," he says.

The polys lower HDLs, but they

Go-for-It Guacamole

The key to great-tasting guacamole is a very ripe avocado—but not too ripe. Choose one that's almost black and slightly soft to the touch. Guacamole is best if prepared just before serving.

1	cup chopped ripe avocados
1	cup peeled, seeded and diced tomatoes
¼	cup nonfat yogurt
¼	cup minced scallions
1–3	tablespoons minced fresh coriander
2	teaspoons lime juice
1–3	teaspoons chili powder

In a large bowl, mix the avocados, tomatoes, yogurt, scallions, coriander, lime juice and chili powder until blended but not smooth.

Makes 12 servings.

Per serving: 47 calories, 4 g. fat (73% of calories), 1 g. dietary fiber, 0 mg. cholesterol, 9 mg. sodium.

help lower LDLs at the same time. Monounsaturated fats, on the other hand, have a big bonus: They help lower LDLs ("bad" cholesterol) without affecting the artery-scouring HDLs ("good" cholesterol). One of the best diets in the world, researchers have learned from population studies, is the Mediterranean diet. Greeks and southern Italians, for instance, cook with lots of olive oil, and that means they're getting a bountiful supply of monos in their diet. The result is a much lower rate of heart disease.

And here are some ways to get more monos in your diet.

Make it Greek to you. One of the single best sources of monounsaturated fats is olive oil, the staple of the Mediterranean diet. "It's always best to use as little oil as possible, but if you're going to use cooking oil, olive oil is one alternative," says University of Massachu-

setts heart researcher Dr. Nicolosi.

"Results from a number of studies indicate that when saturated fats are replaced with monounsaturated vegetable oils, such as olive oil, LDLs drop without reducing the HDLs," says Dr. Nicolosi.

In one study, women who switched to olive oil from another type of cooking oil experienced HDL increases of 30 percent after six months. And men who were on a diet that was high in olive oil had a 17 percent boost in their "good" cholesterol.

Two other very good sources of monounsaturated fats are canola oil and peanut oil.

Scuttle the shortening. Olive oil isn't the only trade-off at the kitchen counter. Any kind of unsaturated oil is better than the traditional American skillet-fats such as butter, lard and vegetable shortening.

"Every American over the age of two should be eating less total fat, less saturated fat and more polyunsaturated fat," says Dr. Milani. You'll be helping your cholesterol count every time you substitute safflower oil, sunflower oil, walnut oil, wheat germ oil or corn oil for the old standbys. All of these oils are high in polyunsaturates, so they are definitely better than other cooking fats—although they're not quite as good as olive, peanut and canola oils.

Avoid the tropics. On the other hand, there are certain oils that you should definitely avoid. The overall worst is coconut oil, one of the so-called tropical oils used in baked goods like cookies, crackers and cakes: It gets 89 percent of its calories from saturated fats and contains almost no monounsaturated and polyunsaturated fats.

While it's unlikely that you'll cook with tropical oils, you'll certainly find them if you look on food labels: Products containing the tropicals are high in saturated fats. Other cooking oils and fats to avoid include cottonseed oil, vegetable shortening, chicken fat and lard.

Get hooked on fish. Some fish are

GO CRAZY OVER NUTS

A handful of nuts each day may be all that's needed to keep a handle on high cholesterol. A six-year study of 31,000 men and women already living a heart-healthy lifestyle (they were vegetarians and didn't smoke) found that those who consumed peanuts, almonds, hazelnuts or walnuts at least five times a week had half the risk of heart attack compared to those who ate none.

The secret: The nuts they ate are high in polyunsaturated fats, which have been found to lower levels of LDL, the so-called bad cholesterol.

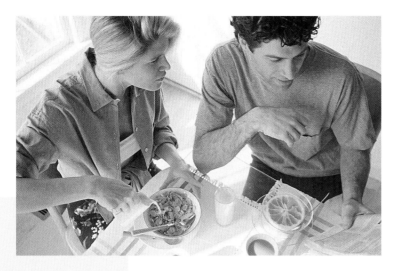

KICK OUT CHOLESTEROL WITH BREAKFAST

Mom nagged you about breakfast so you'd have something that stuck to your ribs—not your blood. The reason that most heart attacks occur between 7:00 A.M. and noon is because that's when blood cells called platelets are "stickiest"—and the stickier your platelets, the greater the chance of clots forming.

And now we have another reason to respect our breakfast obligation. In a study of 12,000 breakfast skippers, researchers found that people who skip breakfast have the highest cholesterol.

While any breakfast is better than nothing, cereal seems to be the heart-smart choice: Cereal eaters have lower cholesterol levels than those who choose another morning meal.

very high in fat, but their fat includes a hefty portion of monos. Mackerel, sablefish, herring, sockeye salmon, catfish, carp and shad are all rich in monos. Some also contain the beneficial omega-3 fatty acids that help protect against heart disease.

Beat the spread. Some margarine can be a heart-healthier alternative to butter. Margarine contains no cholesterol, and it's higher in monounsaturated and polyunsaturated fats than butter.

When choosing a margarine, go with a tub or "soft" type instead of a stick. The reason is that soft or liquid margarines tend to have less saturated fat than regular margarine. Since they're also easier to spread, you can add just a thin layer and you'll be able to eat less in each serving.

Generally, the softer the margarine is, the less it has been processed—and studies have shown that consuming processed vegetable oils increases the risk of heart disease.

SPECIAL TACTICS TO ATTACK PLAQUE

Since managing cholesterol is so important to heart health, researchers have looked at many lifestyle factors to find out what can lower LDLs or raise HDLs. While research shows that nothing can take the place of eating right, here are some recent findings that could help give the brush-off to artery plaque.

Get your partner involved. Give your heart to the person you gave your heart to. Researchers at the University of Nebraska in Omaha found that people are more successful at lowering cholesterol levels when they get their spouse involved in learning the perils of fat and cholesterol, as well as following a healthful diet.

"The encouragement and reassurance a spouse can provide may help people maintain the diet changes in the long run," says Kaye Stanek, Ph.D., associate professor of nutritional science and dietetics at the university.

Take garlic to heart. It appears that this pungent vegetable scares off more than just vampires. Garlic seems to inhibit the production of cholesterol in the liver, says Yu-Yan Yeh, Ph.D., associate professor of nutrition at Pennsylvania State University, who specializes in the study of garlic.

You may see some LDL lowering with as little as two cloves daily, but for the 15 percent reduction shown in his studies, Dr. Yeh recommends eating between five and seven cloves a day.

Keep tabs on your meds. Doctors have found that some prescription medications can force the body to produce excess amounts of cholesterol. If you're taking medication regularly, be sure to ask your doctor whether it has the potential to raise your cholesterol levels. In addition, your doctor might be able to lower your dosage, just to make sure that LDL levels don't go sky-high.

Stay tuned to time-of-life changes. "It's very common for cholesterol levels to increase once a woman goes through menopause," says Dr. Milani. "That's because of the protective characteristics of estrogen, which tends to raise HDLs and lower LDLs. When it's absent, the opposite seems to happen—so women face a greater risk of heart disease after age 50."

Doctors recommend that women pay special attention to their cholesterol during menopause. It's especially important to have more frequent checkups and to stay on a diet that's low in fat.

And there is yet another reason why it's particularly important for menopausal women to follow a low-fat diet, as explained by heart researcher Dr. Denke of the AHA's Nutrition Committee: "Menopause is also associated with weight gain, which may cause higher cholesterol levels. And in general, the heavier you are, the lower your HDL levels and the higher your LDL levels."

Stay on the moderate side of indulgence. No doubt you've heard that you can improve your cholesterol numbers by drinking a glass or two of wine, beer or liquor each night. "But that's not to say you should start drinking for cholesterol health," says Arthur Klatsky, M.D., chief of cardiology at Kaiser Permanente Medical Center in Oakland and a leading researcher on the effects of alcohol on cardiovascular health. "If you are a light-to-moderate drinker, there's no reason to stop, but don't start drinking in an effort to improve your cholesterol."

Alcohol in any form is loaded with calories, so it can contribute to weight gain. And the additional risk that comes with obesity is far greater than any benefits you might get from alcohol. In addition, if you are drinking under your doctor's supervision, take it easy: While moderate drinkers often have lower LDL cholesterol levels than teetotalers, these levels might increase among those who have three drinks or more a day. "Besides, heavy drinking poses other health problems that might be even worse than high cholesterol," Dr. Klatsky cautions.

HERE'S TO YOUR HEALTH

The news on booze is usually anything but something to toast. But after 40 years of research, there seems to be 100 percent proof that moderate drinking boosts the production of artery-scouring HDLs. Compared to teetotalers, people who regularly drink a couple of glasses of wine or beer (or two shots of liquor) lower their risk of death from coronary heart disease by about one-third.

Researchers aren't sure why, but alcohol raises HDLs—sometimes nearly as much as moderate exercise raises them. "There's nothing magical about red wine, even though some people think so," says cardiologist Dr. Arthur Klatsky of Kaiser Permanente Medical Center. "It's the ethyl alcohol—found in any type of alcoholic drink."

As shown by the findings in recent studies (summarized in the graph at right), moderate drinkers have lower heart disease death rates than nondrinkers. But having three or more daily glasses of wine, beer or hard liquor increases that risk.

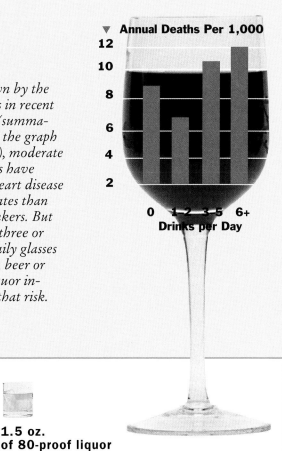

▼ **Annual Deaths Per 1,000**

12
10
8
6
4
2

0 1-2 3-5 6+
Drinks per Day

12 oz.
of beer

=

4–5 oz.
of wine

=

1.5 oz.
of 80-proof liquor

Foods to Beat High Blood Pressure and Stroke

People once thought high blood pressure affected only stressed-out executives trapped in high-pressure jobs. You know, those hard-driving bosses who blow steam from their ears at the drop of a hat.

But now, doctors say, whether you sweat on Wall Street or lounge on Easy Street, you can still get high blood pressure. "Some people with elevated blood pressures are as cool, calm and collected as can be. It's not just the high-strung executive with the cup of coffee in one hand who is affected," says Philip Altus, M.D., professor of medicine at the University of South Florida College of Medicine in Tampa.

You can get high blood pressure no matter what your sex, age, profession or stress level, doctors emphasize. It doesn't matter whether you're a mild-mannered monk or a hot-tempered grouch—everyone is susceptible to this equal-opportunity disease.

High blood pressure, also called hypertension, is one of the most common conditions doctors treat, affecting more than 50 million Americans, or roughly one of every four adults. Unfortunately, it has no cure. And to make things worse, for the majority of people it typically causes no visible symptoms—until you have a stroke or some other conditions directly related to high blood pressure. "It's one of those diseases you have to keep an eye on," Dr. Altus says.

CAN YOU SEE IT COMING?

Doctors aren't sure what causes high blood pressure, although a wide range of factors—including diet—appear to play a large role. And if the condition is left untreated, it can lead to a host of problems related to your heart and circulatory system.

Just for starters, you should know whether you're in one of the higher-risk groups. Risk estimates are based on several factors, including race, age, gender and family history. Consider these facts.

- Blood pressure generally rises with age. Among men and women aged 30 to 39, 11 percent have high blood pressure. That jumps to 64 percent for people aged 70 to 79.
- Young and middle-aged men are more likely to develop high blood pressure than young women. But after middle age, the risks reverse. When women reach menopause—usually in their late forties to early fifties—they are more likely than men of the same age to get high blood pressure.
- People in lower income groups who have less education tend to have higher blood pressure than those who are more affluent or better educated.
- Blacks generally have higher blood pressure than whites.

But whether you're in a high-risk group or not, most doctors agree that you should have your blood pressure

What Is High Blood Pressure?

Blood pressure is the force blood creates while coursing through your arteries. As your heart contracts, it pushes blood out and stiffens the elastic arteries like water surging through a hose. Without this pressure, your body's 60,000-mile network of blood vessels would hang as limp as overcooked spaghetti.

High blood pressure—what doctors call hypertension—refers to the stress placed on arteries, says Dr. George Webb, associate professor specializing in hypertension at the University of Vermont. The excess pressure can lead to thickening of the arteries, heart disease, kidney disease, stroke, the rupture of blood vessels and a variety of other problems.

18 FAT-FIGHTING DIETS TO SCRUB YOUR ARTERIES CLEAN

checked regularly. People with normal blood pressure should be tested every two years. People with a high-normal reading or people at risk should be tested annually.

MUNCHIES AS MUNITIONS

In more than 90 percent of the cases, experts don't know what causes high blood pressure. But they do know what makes it better and worse, and your best weapons may be in your kitchen. A healthy diet and lifestyle should be your first line of defense, Dr. Altus says.

"That's theoretically what most physicians are supposed to prescribe to start," he says. The problem is, doctors have many patients who don't comply with diet and lifestyle recommendations.

Also, it's not just a matter of raiding the refrigerator for solutions. While proper nutrition helps fight high blood pressure, you can't just eat yourself healthy. Battling high blood pressure also means achieving and maintaining your ideal weight, exercising regularly and drinking alcohol only in moderation or not at all.

And for those on blood pressure medication, diet and lifestyle factors are still important. In fact, medication often becomes more effective when people follow dietary guidelines as well, according to Andrew Weil, M.D., associate director for the Division of Social Perspectives in Medicine at the University of Arizona College of Medicine in Tucson.

"I have seen some people who have been able to stop using high blood pressure medicine entirely and others who could reduce their dosage," says Dr. Weil.

SITTING PRETTY WITH POTASSIUM

Start your dietary fight against hypertension with potassium, suggests George D. Webb, Ph.D., associate professor in the Department of Molecular Physiology and Biophysics at the University of Vermont College of Medicine in Burlington.

The importance of potassium has been proven in studies showing that the more of this common mineral you have in your diet, the lower your blood pressure is likely to be. In a large-scale study called INTERSALT, research showed that of 10,079 people studied in 32 countries, those who had the highest amounts of potassium in their bodies had the lowest blood pressure. Those who had the least potassium, on the other hand, were most likely to have high blood pressure. "I think it's pretty well estab-

UPS AND DOWNS OF BLOOD PRESSURE

Doctors express blood pressure in two numbers: systolic and diastolic. The numbers represent how many one-millimeter increments your pressure raises the mercury in a sphygmomanometer (a blood pressure machine). A reading of 120, for example, means your blood pressure raised the mercury 120 millimeters. Readings are expressed as systolic "over" diastolic, and doctors consider both readings significant when measuring blood pressure.

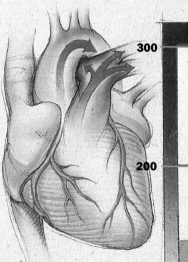

Systolic, the first and larger number, measures what happens when your heart contracts and forces blood through your arteries, creating pressure. A healthy systolic reading is below 140.

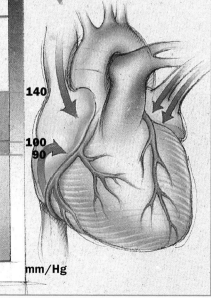

Diastolic, the second, smaller number, measures pressure exerted when your heart expands—that is, when it fills with blood between contractions. A healthy diastolic reading is around 90 or below.

300
200
140
100
90

mm/Hg

lished that potassium lowers blood pressure," Dr. Webb says.

One of potassium's greatest benefits is its ability to rid the body of sodium. The more potassium you eat, the more sodium your body gets rid of, and that's a big boost for your system—which needs to keep sodium under control in order to keep blood pressure at reasonable levels.

True, too much potassium can spell trouble, researchers have found, but it's almost impossible to overdose on potassium if you're getting it from food. You'd have to eat the dietary equivalent of 21 baked potatoes every day to experience some of the negative effects. That's why most experts agree that naturally increasing potassium through diet is a good, safe idea. "As long as you get it in natural foods and don't go on an eating binge, I don't think you can get too much potassium," Dr. Webb says.

An ideal potassium target is 3,500 milligrams—the Daily Value (DV) set by the Food and Drug Administration and the Food Safety and Inspection Service of the U.S. Department of Agriculture. While that's an ambitious goal—you'd have to eat seven or eight bananas to approach that—doctors say whatever foods you eat to get potassium are a plus. Here are some of the shortcuts to more potassium.

Let fruit grow on you. In addition to eating bananas, go for other fresh fruits like peaches and apricots, which are not only good sources of natural potassium but also supply ample amounts of fiber. Aim for two to four servings a day. A serving can consist of ½ cup of sliced fresh fruit or one banana or orange.

Get spud wiser. Potatoes are generous contributors of potassium, but many people avoid them in the belief that they're fattening. Spuds aren't—but what

Best Potassium Bets

When it comes to potassium, the more you get in your food, the better.

Studies have shown that the minimal daily range of potassium is between 1,600 and 2,000 milligrams, or a bit more than you'd get from a couple of potatoes. But the Daily Value is set at 3,500 milligrams, and if you're watching your blood pressure, you should be sure to get at least that.

Fortunately, you don't have to be Sherlock Holmes to find potassium-rich food. Just target your snacks and meals in the right direction.

Food	Portion	Potassium (mg.)
Potato, baked	1	844
Prune juice, canned	8 oz.	704
Adzuki beans, boiled	½ cup	612
Avocado	½	602
Nonfat yogurt	1 cup	578
Clams, steamed	20 small	565
Seedless raisins	½ cup	545
Carrot juice	6 oz.	538
Cantaloupe, cubed	1 cup	494
Dried apricots	10 halves	482
Lima beans, boiled	½ cup	478
Low-fat yogurt	1 cup	468
Yams, cubed, boiled	½ cup	455
Banana	1	451
Acorn squash, baked	½ cup	446
Orange juice	8 oz.	432
Skim milk	8 oz.	405
Trout, baked or broiled	3 oz.	393
Haddock, baked or broiled	3 oz.	339
Sirloin steak, fat trimmed	3 oz.	270

TOP THIS!

Not only are potatoes the best source of potassium, they're excellent sources of complex carbohydrates, which provide long-lasting energy. But we need alternatives to the fat-filled toppings that often get glopped on top. Sour cream, cheddar cheese and bacon bits may taste good—but there's no reason to add that fat to a potato.

Instead, here are some healthier, low-fat toppings to enhance the tantalizing taste of your tuber.

◾ *Instead of sour cream, opt for plain low-fat or nonfat yogurt.*

◾ *Choose a salsa of your choice—mild to hot—to wake up your palate.*

◾ *Squeeze some lemon juice onto the potato and sprinkle it with black pepper.*

◾ *Say cheese with low-fat Monterey Jack or cottage cheese.*

◾ *Try chopped tomatoes, jalapeño peppers, shredded spinach, mushrooms or steamed broccoli.*

goes on top of that freshly baked Idaho potato can be a major menace because of the fat. If you're in the habit of adding sour cream, butter and bacon bits to potatoes, you're adding unnecessary fat to a prime source of health-rendering potassium. Change your topping style, and spuds take the cake as potassium-rich foods.

If you favor boiled potatoes over baked potatoes, here's a clue to potassium preservation: For maximum effect, steam potatoes rather than boiling them, since boiling depletes the potassium. Just place the potatoes in a steaming basket and put the basket in a large saucepan with about an inch of water. Cover, bring the water to a boil and steam for 10 to 15 minutes.

Choose nuts. Nuts are good sources of potassium, and they're also high in fiber, which makes them good for snacking. But since many nuts are also high in fat, you don't want to go overboard. For a potassium pick-me-up, have no more than a handful of pistachios (which have more potassium than most other kinds of nuts). Or buy ½ pound of chestnuts (low in fat, high in potassium) and roast some in the oven. Just be sure to cut an *X* in the shell first so they don't explode. Then roast them on a baking sheet at 425°F for 15 to 20 minutes.

CALCIUM: IT DOES THE BODY GOOD

Numerous parents have encouraged their kids to chug down milk. But now we know that adults, too, can benefit from milk and milk products.

The reason: Milk contains a big cargo of calcium, and researchers think that calcium is a major player in reducing high blood pressure. In a 13-year California study sponsored by the National Center for Health Statistics, researchers examined 6,634 men and women to find out how they reacted to increased calcium in their diet. They concluded that people who consumed one gram of calcium a day—the amount in two cups of nonfat yogurt—were able to lower their

risk of high blood pressure by an average of 12 percent.

While these results have not been entirely supported by other studies, many experts believe that calcium, for some, can have a beneficial effect on blood pressure. Just how? Theories vary. Some researchers say calcium induces a hormonal change that affects blood pressure. Others claim it affects the smooth muscle cells in blood vessels, causing them to relax and expand, thus allowing greater blood flow.

Even though we don't have the final word on calcium and high blood pressure, most experts agree you should at least get your DV of 1,000 milligrams. And there are some doctors, like Dr. Weil, who suggest taking up to 1,500 milligrams a day. One caution, however: If you're prone to kidney stones, you'll want to avoid upping the calcium in your diet too much, because it can contribute to stones in some people.

Of course, another benefit of calcium, particularly for women, is its ability to stave off osteoporosis, a decrease in bone mass and density that can weaken bones and affect posture.

With all the pluses calcium contains for your blood pressure and overall health, why wait? Here's how to get more in your diet.

Have a moo-ving experience. Since dairy products are high in calcium, go to the source—good old-fashioned milk. Dr. Altus advises drinking low-fat or skim milk. "That takes the fat out, but leaves the calcium in," he says.

One eight-ounce glass of skim milk or 1 percent low-fat milk contains about 300 milligrams of calcium. Some other calcium-rich dairy products are low-fat yogurt, Swiss and cheddar cheese and frozen yogurt.

Say *hola* to tortillas. Give a hearty *bienvenidos* ("welcome") to lime-processed tortillas, which are prepared following a traditional Mexican recipe. In the Mexican-style lime processing, corn kernels are soaked in lime-enriched water. When made this way, the tortillas become an ex-

EAT MORE POTASSIUM, TAKE FEWER PILLS

Even when a doctor prescribes medication to control blood pressure, diet still counts . . . a lot! In fact, some people with high blood pressure have found that a potassium-rich diet and healthy lifestyle avert the need for medicine. Consider this:

In a study at the Second Medical School at the University of Naples in Italy, 28 of 54 adults on blood pressure medication increased their potassium an average of 50 percent by eating fruits, vegetables and legumes. The remaining 26 kept to their normal diet. After a year, 9 of the 26 in the potassium group could stop taking medication, compared to 2 in the nonpotassium group.

Overall, 21 of the 26 members of the high-potassium group could use less than half the medication they were previously using. Only 6 people in the nonpotassium group could do this.

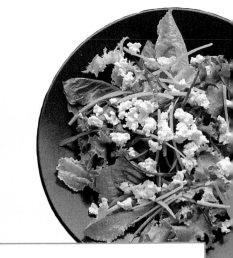

The Joy of Soy

What does tofu, the custardlike soybean curd that's the protein favorite of many vegetarians, taste like? It's hard to say, because tofu changes flavor to mimic other foods it's cooked with, much like a chameleon changes color to match its background.

This chameleon totes a ton of calcium—517 milligrams (more than half a day's supply) in just a cup. It's also high in protein, low in saturated fat and calories and relatively inexpensive. You can find tofu in the produce section of most supermarkets, sold in 10- to 16-ounce containers and packaged with a small amount of water. After opening, store any unused tofu in an airtight container with enough fresh water to cover it. Change the water daily, and rinse the tofu before use. Kept this way, it will stay fresh for up to two weeks.

PUT THE SQUEEZE ON YOUR TOFU

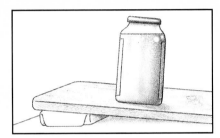

You can press tofu so it will retain its shape during cooking. Wrap it in absorbent paper, then position a cutting board on top at an angle. Put a weight (a heavy jar, for instance) on top of the board and let it stand until the water oozes out—usually about half an hour.

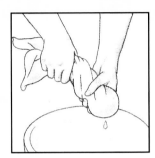

Here's a quick way to squeeze out the water to make crumbly tofu. Put it in a dish towel, twist the towel's ends and wring dry.

TASTY TOFU TIPS

In some parts of the world, tofu is served as often as french fries are served in America—and with good reason. It's fast, filling, versatile and delicious. And here's how to make this calcium-packed food into an enhancer of many all-American meals.

- *Use it as a quick meat substitute. Combine crumbled tofu with ground beef for more healthful meat loaf.*
- *Use chunks in spaghetti sauce.*
- *Crumble it up and add to scrambled eggs or egg salad.*
- *Mix it with peanut butter when making peanut butter and jelly sandwiches.*
- *Crumble it and sprinkle on salads.*
- *Mix it in a blender and add to soups for creamy texture.*

cellent source of calcium. Just compare the 44 milligrams of calcium found in an average corn tortilla to the 27 milligrams in a slice of white bread.

Eat your vegetables. Seems that moms do know best, especially when it comes to calcium. Green leafy vegetables, such as spinach, with 244 milligrams of calcium per one-cup serving, are good sources.

Lose the booze. Some scientists believe alcohol inhibits calcium absorption and increases its excretion. Many doctors say it's fine to have a drink or two a day, and this amount of alcohol may even help your blood pressure. But if you're not getting much calcium in your diet, you might want to steer clear of beer and other alcoholic drinks.

Have a bone to pick on. Soft bones are full of calcium, so eat sardines or canned salmon, which have lots of chewable bones.

SCUTTLE THE SODIUM

Calling salt's role in blood pressure controversial is like calling Romeo and Juliet just another love story. In fact, some people believe that if a nuclear holocaust struck, the only things to survive would be cockroaches and the long-standing medical debate on salt.

For the record, sodium is not salt. Sodium is a naturally occurring mineral. Salt is a compound composed of sodium and chloride. Yet the words salt and

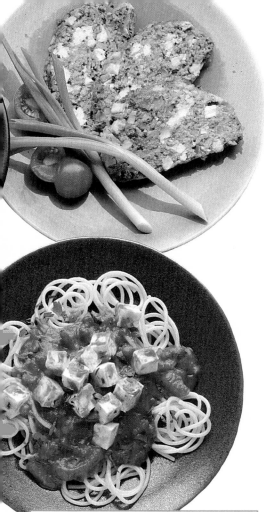

sodium sometimes are used interchangeably because salt contains 40 percent sodium.

But whether the discussion is about salt or sodium, it all returns to the same question: How important is this mineral in the diet?

Like potassium and calcium, sodium plays an important role in the human body. It aids in the transmission of nerve impulses, assists in muscle contraction, maintains blood volume and regulates cell fluid levels. While there may be many other factors that balance out the effect of sodium, there's no question that it's a powerfully influential mineral.

But sodium has its drawbacks, too—especially in large quantities. Some experts say sodium is your ticket to the blood pressure blues. Just for starters, sodium can cause fluid retention. When your body soaks up more fluid and releases less, the buildup of volume results in higher blood pressure. Doctors who blame sodium for high blood pressure say it also can have another damaging effect: The sodium can settle into arterial muscle cells and spark a chemical reaction that results in raised blood pressure.

On the flip side of the debate are the experts who say that sodium has gotten a bum rap—that the real issue is your sodium sensitivity. Studies have shown that some people are less sensitive to salt—and reducing it may have little effect on their blood pressure. And for others, reducing salt may actually be harmful, so be sure to check with your doctor before cutting it completely out of your diet.

But even though the debate continues—and new studies are being done every year—"no one believes a whole lot of salt is good for you," Dr. Altus says. "No one's advocating giving everyone free use of the salt shaker."

But in this whole debate one thing is clear: Americans consume too much. And people who are sodium sensitive stand a good chance of lowering their blood pressure if they reduce their consumption of the salt that comes from the

CALCIUM COMPARISONS	
Food	Calcium (mg.)
Tofu, firm 1 cup	517
Yogurt, nonfat 1 cup	452
Fruit yogurt, low-fat 1 cup	345
Sardines (with bones) 3 oz.	325
Milk, skim 1 cup	302
Swiss cheese 1 oz.	269
Spinach, cooked 1 cup	245
Cheddar cheese 1 oz.	202
Oysters 1 cup	202
Tapioca pudding (made with 2% milk) ½ cup	149

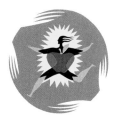

BREAKTHROUGHS IN HEALING

1896

Italian physician Scipione Riva-Rocci invents a portable blood pressure machine that serves as a prototype for today's models.

1930–50

Researchers realize that high blood pressure—once considered just a symptom of hardening of the arteries—is by itself a complex and dangerous medical condition. Implication: Dietary changes that lower blood pressure also increase life expectancy.

1987

The Honolulu Heart Study finds magnesium—more than any other nutrient—is associated with low blood pressure in 615 men. Doctors encourage increased magnesium in the American diet.

1988

Massive INTERSALT study by the INTERSALT Cooperative Research Group confirms earlier studies showing high blood pressure associated with high salt intake. Based on the findings in this study—which includes 10,079 people in 32 countries—most doctors recommend reduced-sodium diets for all those with high blood pressure.

shaker, as well as sodium from other sources.

Average Americans typically consume 4,000 to 5,800 milligrams or more of sodium a day, far more than the recommended 2,400-milligram limit. And a lot of that extra amount is just soaked up by the body. Since we excrete only about 115 milligrams a day, most of us are taking in thousands of milligrams of extra sodium. Yet we need only a scant 500 milligrams a day to survive—so the extra doses are traveling around, just looking for trouble.

There are no proven benefits of extra sodium, and there are certainly many drawbacks for people whose blood pressure reacts to it. Since cutting back is the best route to take, here's how.

Take it without a grain of salt. The salt shaker is a standard monolith on most American tables, but like some other monuments to past eating habits, you're free to ignore it. And you should, according to John G. Gums, Pharm.D., associate professor of pharmacy and medicine at the University of Florida in Gainesville.

"Next time you go to a restaurant, observe," says Dr. Gums. "You'll notice three types of people. Some will sit down and never look for a shaker. Some will eat a few bites, then reach for a shaker. Then there's the third type. These are the people who won't even sit down until they have a shaker."

Dr. Gums encourages everyone to shake the habit of looking for the salt. Some people find they enjoy the natural flavor of food more without salt. But if you need more flavor, Dr. Gums says, reach for the spice rack rather than the salt shaker.

Kick the can. Avoid canned and processed foods. Manufacturers add lots of sodium during processing, and most foods already contain natural sodium.

In a study by the Rowett Research Institute at Bucksburn in Aberdeen, Scotland, researchers traced salt in various foods by using a chemical marker. They discovered that 75 percent of daily salt intake came from the salt added in the processing of foods, while only 10 percent of daily salt intake came from the natural sodium found in foods. That means that even though canned soups and other processed foods don't necessarily taste salty, they're stocked with trouble for anyone prone to high blood pressure.

Don't cull the crullers. Pastries, though tasty, are high in sodium. A standard cake-type doughnut contains 291 milligrams of artery-abusing sodium, or about 31 potato chips' worth. A cheese Danish has 319 milligrams of sodium, and a fruit Danish is worse—it has 333 milligrams. That's about two-thirds of what our bodies need each day.

Go for a salt substitute. If you crave the taste of salt and can't shake the shaker, try a salt substitute. Most of these readily available substitutes are made of potassium chloride, which will help boost your potassium while lowering your sodium intake.

"When you use potassium chloride on food it tastes as salty as salt, but it has

2 = 119

cups of cottage cheese with 2 stalks of celery   **potato chips**

no sodium," Dr. Gums says.

One well-known brand is Morton Lite Salt. It tastes like salt, and $\frac{1}{6}$ teaspoon (one serving) contains a mere 190 milligrams of sodium, as opposed to 333 milligrams per serving of ordinary salt. And each teaspoon of Lite Salt contains a respectable 260 milligrams of potassium.

Drive past the drive-through. Yes, it's inexpensive and convenient, but eating fast food is a fast way of overloading on sodium. Consider a McDonald's six-piece Chicken McNugget lunch. It has 580 milligrams of sodium. And a hamburger? The Burger King Double Whopper with cheese, for instance, packs 1,340 milligrams. That's not including french fries, which generally have 124 milligrams of sodium per serving.

Read voraciously. Read labels on everything you eat and become familiar with the sodium content of your favorite foods. Check packages, cans, frozen foods and soft drinks. You can even find out how much sodium is in fast food.

Next time you eat at a fast-food restaurant, just ask for a list of foods and ingredients. (Sometimes the list is posted.)

By reading labels, you'll discover, for example, that the all-American hot dog contains 670 milligrams of salt—the equivalent of about 70 potato chips. And if you add mustard or sauerkraut, then you're on a real salt binge: Combined, they have as much or more sodium than the hot dog.

Sideline sodium sauces. Salad dressings can be the high road to high blood pressure. At home, you can use low-sodium dressings, but how can you combat sodium overload when you're eating out? A creamy-tasting dressing can add several hundred milligrams of sodium to your meal.

Don't let the chef push your blood pressure around. Instead, ask for dressings to be served on the side. That way, you can pour on enough for flavor without pouring on the sodium.

Regular French dressing, for example, contains 427 milligrams of sodium per two-tablespoon serving. Your salad will taste just as good with half that amount—and you'll cut your sodium intake by more than 210 milligrams.

Eat your vegetables—again! As far as high blood pressure goes, you're doing your arteries a favor every time you choose vegetables, which are high in nutrients and low in sodium. The key, though, is to serve them without a dash of salt.

SURREPTITIOUS SODIUM SOURCES

Sodium can hide where you'd never expect to find it. Many of us know, for example, that regular potato chips are very high in sodium. But look at the list below and you'll find that every food but celery is *higher* in sodium than a serving of potato chips. Here are 13 common sources of sodium that might surprise you.

Food	Portion	Sodium (mg.)
Sauerkraut, canned	*1 cup*	*1,561*
Potato salad	*1 cup*	*1,323*
Vegetable soup, canned	*1 cup*	*1,010*
Dill pickle, large	*1*	*833*
Cheese pizza	*2 slices*	*672*
Cottage cheese	*½ cup*	*459*
Tomato juice, canned or bottled	*4 oz.*	*441*
Total cereal	*1 oz.*	*352*
White or wheat bread	*2 slices*	*268*
Green peas, canned, drained	*½ cup*	*186*
Skim milk	*8 oz.*	*126*
Potato chips	*¾ oz.*	*100*
Chopped celery	*½ cup*	*52*

MORE MAGNESIUM, PLEASE

Like a fledgling actor in community theater, magnesium plays many roles in the body. In fact, this silvery-white mineral, in microscopic amounts, participates in more than 300 chemical reactions that help keep us alive. About 40 percent of our body's magnesium lies in muscle and soft tissue. Along with calcium, it's one of nature's anti-stress agents. Some experts think it relaxes muscles in the blood vessel walls, allowing blood to flow through more easily.

MIX IT UP WITH SPICES

Just because you're steering clear of sodium doesn't mean your food has to be tasteless. Your supermarket's spice shelf abounds with hot, tart, aromatic and tantalizing flavors that can easily replace salt. Mixed together, these spices can enhance the flavors of your favorite foods far more than table salt.

Here are some spice mixtures you can make in minutes. Sprinkle them on during cooking, or have them ready at the table for fish, fowl and everything in between. Just mix the ingredients and store in a three-ounce spice container. These spice mixtures will keep almost indefinitely as long as they stay dry.

Although magnesium research continues, some studies show this ubiquitous mineral is an effective high blood pressure fighter. Consider the following:

■ In one of the largest magnesium studies ever, researchers at Harvard Medical School and Brigham and Women's Hospital in Boston evaluated diet and blood pressure in 58,218 women. They found that women who ate a diet with more magnesium also had lower blood pressure.

■ In the Honolulu Heart Study at the Kuakini Medical Center in Hawaii, doctors examined the effects of 61 nutritional factors on high blood pressure. After examining 615 Hawaiian men, they found that high magnesium—more than any other nutrient—meant lower blood pressure.

The Egg Enhancer
(for all egg dishes)
1 tsp. dried parsley
1 tsp. dried basil
1 tsp. dried chervil
1 tsp. dried chives
1 tsp. dried marjoram
1 tsp. dried tarragon
Makes 2 Tbsp.

Chicken-Lickin' Spices
(good on all poultry)
2 tsp. dried chervil
2 tsp. garlic powder
2 tsp. dried tarragon
Makes 2 Tbsp.

Tart 'n' Peppery Shake-On (for all foods)
2 tsp. dried basil
2 tsp. dried marjoram
2 tsp. paprika
2 tsp. dried thyme
1 tsp. powdered ginger
½ tsp. dried lemon peel
¼ tsp. dry mustard
⅛ tsp. dried sage
⅛ tsp. cayenne pepper
Makes about 3 Tbsp.

Flavor for Fish
(a special blend for seafood)
2 tsp. dried chives
2 tsp. celery seed
2 tsp. dried dill
Makes 2 Tbsp.

Savory All-Purpose Blend (for all foods)
1 Tbsp. dried basil
2 tsp. celery seed
2 tsp. dried savory
1 tsp. dried thyme
1 tsp. dried marjoram
Makes 3 Tbsp.

The Beef Booster
(for steak and hamburger)
2 tsp. dried parsley
2 tsp. garlic powder
2 tsp. onion powder
2 tsp. ground black pepper
Makes about 3 Tbsp.

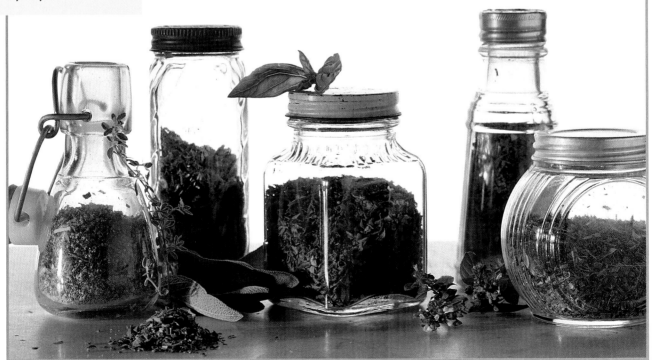

With such encouraging evidence, you'd think people would chug magnesium like beer and pretzels on Super Bowl Sunday. But they don't. In fact, without knowing it, people are turning away from magnesium faster than you can say "first down."

According to the National Research Council, per capita magnesium consumption declined 20 percent between 1909 and 1985. It's generally recognized that most people, especially women, don't get as much magnesium as they need, says Dr. Gums. He recommends 500 milligrams of magnesium for both men and women who are concerned about high blood pressure.

Although too much magnesium can cause diarrhea, it's unlikely you'll ever get too much from food, so here's how to get your magnesium naturally.

Reverse the trend. Since experts think our shrinking magnesium levels are because of our diet, reverse the trend by eating more fiber and unprocessed foods.

Many unprocessed foods—including nuts, legumes and whole grains—naturally contain magnesium. Other good sources are green leafy vegetables that store the mineral in chlorophyll (the pigment that gives them their green color). A half cup of spinach, for instance, contains 78 milligrams of magnesium—and swiss chard has about the same amount. Beet greens contain 49 milligrams per ½ cup, and kale has 37 milligrams. Green peas are also high in magnesium, with about 31 milligrams per ½ cup.

Cut the cantaloupe. Most commonly eaten fruits are not good sources of magnesium, but there are some exceptions—such as bananas, cantaloupe, kiwi and pineapple. One banana, for instance, has 33 milligrams of magnesium.

Supplement your diet. If you just can't get to the produce section often enough, Dr. Gums suggests taking a supplement. He recommends magnesium chloride (such as Slow-Mag), which contains 64 milligrams per tablet. Even though it's available without a pre-scription, you should check with your doctor first.

Can the soda. Phosphates, which are found in soft drinks and come from phosphorus, interfere with magnesium absorption. This happens when the phosphate and magnesium molecules combine, which sometimes occurs because of their opposing electrical charges. This combination is not a match made in heaven, because every time a phosphate meets magnesium, it means less magnesium for your body.

A typical soft drink, for example, might have as much as 75 milligrams of phosphates per 12-ounce bottle. A soda or two shouldn't cause a problem, but you'll get more magnesium if you don't overdo it. So keep this in mind before you stock up on soda. You'll do your arteries a favor.

MAKE TWO THE LIMIT

Doctors have known for decades that alcohol affects the body in many ways, including raising blood pressure.

One of the first studies documenting this came in 1915, when researchers discovered that members of the French military who drank at least three liters of wine a day had higher blood pressures than those who drank less.

While three liters (about ¾ gallon) is enough to pickle a private, the findings still apply: Excess alcohol raises blood pressure.

But alcohol needn't be taboo. Some experts even suggest that moderate drinking may be healthy.

"Alcohol may be beneficial to some people," says the University of Arizona's Dr. Weil. "It can be a stress reliever, and it may be good for your heart and cholesterol." Just remember that two's the limit when it comes to blood pressure. More than two drinks is no longer considered moderate.

MORE THAN JUST J-J-J-JITTERS

For many of us, the first order of business in the morning, after stumbling out of bed, is to lurch for the coffee pot. Only after a brief rendezvous with Mr. Coffee in the kitchen do we feel that we're we ready to face the world. For many people, these early-morning kitchen encounters are more than habits. They're rituals of sorts.

"We do have our morning rituals, and for many people caffeine certainly is one of them," says William R. Lovallo, Ph.D., professor of psychiatry and behavioral sciences at the University of Oklahoma Health Sciences Center in Oklahoma City.

Caffeine stimulates the body, which in turn raises blood pressure. So if you're watching your blood pressure, it makes sense to limit—or even try to eliminate—this potent beverage from your daily diet, says Dr. Lovallo. Here are his recommendations.

Put some "de" in your "caf." To eliminate the 102 milligrams of caffeine in each average cup of brewed coffee, switch to decaffeinated. This gives you the taste and morning ritual without the caffeine.

Since dropping caffeine can cause withdrawal-like side effects, including headache and lethargy, you should make the switch gradually. If you're a coffee drinker, mix caffeinated and decaffeinated coffee for a few days before going cold turkey.

Take an instant remedy. If you want to reduce your caffeine instead of eliminating it, switch to instant coffee. An average serving of instant coffee contains about half the caffeine of brewed coffee.

Avoid caffeine-rich foods. If you swap a midafternoon cup of coffee for tea, soda or a few chocolate bars, you're still punishing your blood pressure with caffeine.

One can of Mountain Dew, for example, contains 55 milligrams of caffeine—more than half as much as a cup of brewed coffee. A six-ounce cup of regular Lipton tea has between 35 and 50 milligrams of caffeine. And while a typical chocolate bar has much less caffeine,

it's still there. A 1½-ounce bar of milk chocolate, for instance, contains about 9 milligrams.

Tip the Scales in Your Favor

Remember English class, when you were taught the axiom of good writing, "Less is more."?

That aphorism came from 19th-century poet Robert Browning. Little did Browning—or your teachers—realize how nicely this applies to weight and high blood pressure.

Doctors know that a relationship exists between excess weight and high blood pressure. Studies have shown that people who are 30 percent over their ideal weight are more likely to develop high blood pressure than those who are not as overweight.

So the less extra weight you have, the better your chances of avoiding or fighting high blood pressure. And since more than one-quarter of Americans are overweight, nearly everyone's blood pressure will benefit from battling the bulge.

"I think the three dietary elements in regard to blood pressure I would stress are low sodium, high potassium and weight loss, if you're overweight," concludes Dr. Webb of the University of Vermont. "You really need to do all those things, not just one."

Fishing for Answers

So many high blood pressure studies are under way that new developments are reported every year. Some of the studies on high blood pressure and diet point to fish oil and garlic as two foods that may be chock-full of benefits for people prone to the problem.

In 1993, for example, researchers at Johns Hopkins University School of Medicine reported that taking doses of fish oil can lower your blood pressure. Reviewing the results of 17 studies, researchers found that dosages of at least three grams a day—equivalent to about two three-ounce servings of canned pink salmon or three one-gram fish-oil supplements—lowered systolic blood pressure an average of 5.5 points and diastolic an average of 3.5 points.

The research is still preliminary, but some doctors surmise that fish oil's omega-3 polyunsaturated fatty acids affect blood vessel constriction and dilation. These omega-3 fatty acids are found primarily in fish and shellfish. (Among the best sources of fish oil are salmon, tuna and mackerel.)

Other researchers caution against taking this advice hook, line and sinker. They say something's fishy, because other tests, including one by the Center for Research on Health and Aging in Chicago, found that fish oil had no effect on high blood pressure. In the Chicago test, 18 people with mild hypertension were given either fish oil or an olive oil placebo. After 12 weeks, researchers noticed no significant changes in blood pressure.

That study was a small one, however, so the jury is still out on this question. Since fish oil has been shown to help some people—and you might be among them—there's probably nothing wrong with feasting on fish. But you should check with your doctor before taking fish-oil capsules.

GARLIC GOODIES

A number of recent studies have examined the effects of garlic on blood pressure. It's not the first time. Investigators from antiquity to modern times have been intrigued by this pungent herb's potential uses.

Around 1500 B.C., for example, Egyptians ate garlic to combat heart disease. Centuries later, people believed that old folk remedies containing garlic cured "hot blood," a condition that frequently occurred in corpulent people who are now believed to have suffered from high blood pressure.

Modern medical researchers say that garlic advocates just might be on the right track. In one study at the Clinical Research Center in New Orleans, the study participants were given a total of 2,400 milligrams of over-the-counter garlic tablets (eight 300-milligram tablets) per day. The researchers noted that there was a significant drop in their blood pressure.

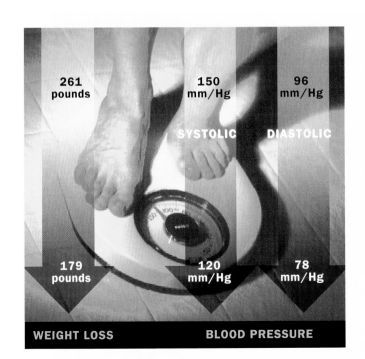

SHED POUNDS—
DROP THE PRESSURE

In 1985, researchers at the University of California pinpointed the connection between weight loss and high blood pressure. Their findings: When overweight people shed their extra pounds, blood pressure plummeted.

In one part of the study, 39 people who were overweight and had high blood pressure were placed on a low-calorie protein diet. Before the diet, their average weight was 261 pounds. Blood pressure averaged 150 over 96.

During the weight-loss phase of the study—which lasted 16 weeks—participants lost, on average, 82 pounds. While shedding these extra pounds, people's blood pressure sank to an average of 120 over 78.

Reverse the Risk of Heart Attack

You've probably heard the story repeated at least a dozen times: How it came out of nowhere, a pain crushing his chest. How she was playing happily with her grandchildren one moment and gasping for air the next.

It happens 171 times every hour of every day—the frantic call to 911, the desperate struggle in the ambulance or emergency room, the tears and prayers for a loved one hit by heart attack. But no matter who the victim is, there's always the shocking disbelief that it "suddenly" and "unexpectedly" happened.

Actually, heart attack doesn't "just happen." Usually it's been years in the making.

"When you compare all the factors that contribute to a heart attack, it seems as though diet is probably the most significant," says Basil Rifkind, M.D., chief of the Lipid Metabolism and Atherogenesis Branch of the National Heart, Lung and Blood Institute in Bethesda, Maryland.

"You look at countries like Japan where people smoke a great deal, have high blood pressure and live with a lot of stress. But they still have a negligible rate of coronary disease because they have much lower blood cholesterol levels," Dr. Rifkind notes. "Once your cholesterol level is high—which results from a diet high in saturated fats and cholesterol—these other factors put you at additional risk for heart disease."

AN INFARCTION IN ACTION

A heart attack is technically called a myocardial infarction. *Myo* means muscle and *cardia* means heart, and an *infarction* occurs when tissue dies because of oxygen starvation. It usually happens when a blood clot lodges in an artery narrowed by fatty deposits of hardened cholesterol—the result of a bad diet. Without blood, cells can't get oxygen and the heart muscle in that area stops working and dies.

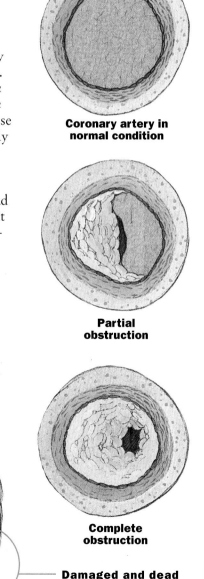

Coronary artery in normal condition

Partial obstruction

Complete obstruction

Damaged and dead heart muscle

A NATION AT RISK?

A quick scan of the overall American diet helps to explain why heart attack is as American as hot dogs and apple pie (both of which are way too high in saturated fat). As many as 1½ million heart attacks occur here each year—and one in three is fatal.

Your chances of having or dying from a heart attack are greater if you are male, are over 65 or have a family history of heart disease. Other factors that increase your risk include smoking, stress, being overweight or having diabetes, high blood pressure or high cholesterol.

If you're already at risk because of one of these factors, a poor diet just adds potential problems—particularly when that diet contributes to obesity, high blood pressure and high cholesterol. But while the way you eat can be a cause of heart attack, researchers are learning that it can also be the cure.

"There have been 11 major studies showing that you can reverse plaque in the arteries, and part of the therapy has been a diet low in saturated fats," says Neil Stone, M.D., associate professor of medicine at Northwestern University School of Medicine in Chicago and chairman of the American Heart Association's (AHA) Nutrition Committee.

In fact, Dr. Stone notes that, in some cases, diet alone may be as effective in reducing heart attack risk as going on a low-fat diet *and* taking cholesterol-lowering medication. "At least one study showed that diet alone could produce a risk regression rate that was similar to what was accomplished previously with diet and medication."

UNCOVERING HIDDEN FATS

So the answer to reversing the risk of heart attack seems obvious enough: Follow the AHA's guidelines of getting no more than 30 percent of your overall calories from fat sources. And, within those guidelines, you need to pay particular attention to which kind of fat you're getting. In order to reduce the risk of

heart attack significantly, no more than 10 percent of your calories should come from saturated fats. Unfortunately, what isn't so obvious is just where all those fat calories come from.

For instance, we're told that saturated fats are associated with the clogging of arteries and can cause heart attack, and these are mostly so-called animal fats. And we're told that vegetable fats, such as monounsaturated fats, can be heart-healthy.

But what we're not always told is that some vegetable fats can do even more damage than animal fats—and many of those fats are no further away than your own kitchen shelves.

TRANS-FORMING YOUR DIET

Trans-fatty acids are the result of a commercial process called hydrogenation, in which cheaper (and usually heart-healthy) vegetable oils are turned into a semisolid state resembling butter. Hundreds of food manufacturers use hydrogenated ingredients to give their foods longer shelf-life, more texture and a richer, more appealing taste. Foods that are most likely to contain trans-fatty acids include fast foods, baked goods, snack foods, sweets and even pizza. But what's good for the palate is nasty for the heart.

"In one study we found a twofold increase in risk of heart attack between people who had the most trans-fatty acids in their diet and those who had the least," says Alberto Ascherio, M.D., Dr.P.H., assistant professor of nutrition and epidemiology at Harvard University School of Public Health. "And other studies have had similar findings."

Some studies indicate that trans-fatty acids may do their dirty work by raising harmful LDLs while possibly lowering helpful HDLs. And apparently trans-fatty acids are worse than saturated fats when it comes to changing the ratio between overall cholesterol and HDL cholesterol. In fact, "they seem to increase the ratio between overall cholesterol levels and HDL cholesterol at twice the

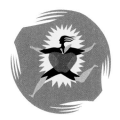

BREAKTHROUGHS IN HEALING

1 9 4 8

The Framingham Heart Study is launched. Over the years, this study of residents of Framingham, Massachusetts, will show that eating a high-fat diet increases risk of heart attack.

1 9 5 7

At 40, inventor Nathan Pritikin is diagnosed with heart disease. He begins eating a low-fat diet and demonstrates that the "Pritikin diet" sharply improves his heart condition. In 1976, he opens the Pritikin Longevity Center in Santa Barbara, California, to help other heart disease patients.

1 9 7 9

Dean Ornish, M.D., publishes his first study finding that heart patients placed on an extremely low-fat diet, along with stress-reducing lifestyle changes, can *reverse* damage done by heart disease.

1 9 9 3

A long-term study finds that patients who eat a low-fat, high-fiber diet and take a placebo (a blank pill) instead of a heart drug lower their risk of heart attack just as much as members of another group on a low-fat diet who take prescription medication.

The Right Mix of Fats

All cooking oils have two things in common: a hefty 120 calories per table-spoon and the fact that every one of those calories comes from fat.

"But some oils are less harmful than others—namely those that are lowest in percentage of saturated fats and highest in monounsaturated and polyunsaturated fats," says University of Massachusetts researcher Dr. Robert Nicolosi. The chart below shows some of the best oils, which are lowest in saturated fat.

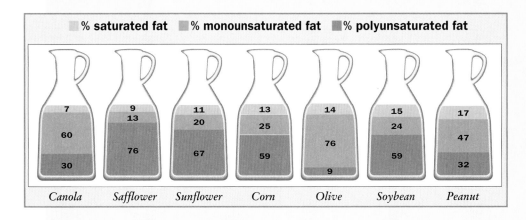

| ■ % saturated fat | ■ % monounsaturated fat | ■ % polyunsaturated fat |

Canola	Safflower	Sunflower	Corn	Olive	Soybean	Peanut
7	9	11	13	14	15	17
60	13	20	25	76	24	47
30	76	67	59	9	59	32

rate of saturated fats," says Lisa Litin, R.D., a research dietitian at Harvard. The more trans-fatty acids you have in your diet, the more your heart disease risk goes up.

The difficulty with trans-fats, as they are called, is in detecting them. "The food industry doesn't want you to be concerned about these, which is why they're not listed on food labels," says Bruce Holub, Ph.D., a researcher and nutritionist at the University of Guelph in Ontario, Canada. "What's really frightening is that in our investigation, we found that the majority of processed and fast foods marketed as being cholesterol free or low in saturated fat are some of the richest sources of trans-fatty acids."

Although there are no guidelines for the amount of trans-fats you should eat, experts believe the fewer, the better. The the typical American, they estimate, consumes approximately 15 "trans" fat grams a day. But it's really not that difficult to shave a number of grams from that daily total. Here's how to tell where the trans-fats come from.

Clue in to warnings. "The best way to detect trans-fatty acids is to know what to look for on food labels," says Dr. Ascherio. "If you see the words *hydrogenated* or *partially hydrogenated vegetable oil,* the food contains trans-fatty acids and consumption should be limited."

Other clues: "Any label that says, 'May contain one or more of the following' and lists partially hydrogenated cottonseed, soybean or other oils indicates it's been chemically changed and contains trans-fatty acids," adds Litin.

Reminder: Food labels list ingredients from highest quantity to lowest. So if you see any of these ingredients among the top three or four on the list, you know the food product is very high in trans-fatty acids. If the hydrogenated fats are lower on the list, then the amount of trans-fatty acids in the product is probably minimal.

Do your math. If you're still not sure, you can do some math to figure out exactly how many trans-fats you're eating. Even though the exact amount of trans-fatty acids is not specified on the

COOKING FATS TO AVOID

The worst cooking fats get 25 percent or more of their calories from saturated fats. They include:

COCONUT OIL
*89% saturated
6% monounsaturated
2% polyunsaturated*

BUTTER
*64% saturated
29% monounsaturated
4% polyunsaturated*

PALM OIL
*50% saturated
36% monounsaturated
9% polyunsaturated*

LARD
*39% saturated
45% monounsaturated
11% polyunsaturated*

COTTONSEED OIL
*26% saturated
18% monounsaturated
53% polyunsaturated*

VEGETABLE SHORTENING
*25% saturated
45% monounsaturated
20% polyunsaturated*

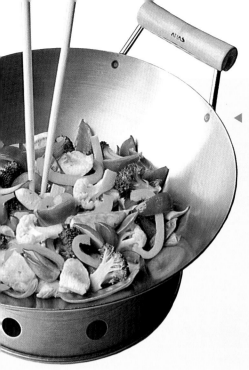

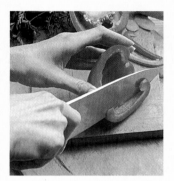

◀ *When you're sautéing vegetables, you should add only a tablespoon of canola, corn or olive oil to keep the vegetables from sticking. If you're cooking dry vegetables like carrots or cauliflower, moisten the frying pan or wok with a mixture of oil and citrus juice.*

Slice your vegetables into big bites ▶ rather than small ones. Small pieces get hotter in the stir-fry, and the high heat depletes nutrients.

THE MANY WONDERS OF OLIVE OIL

For decades, olive oil took a backseat to the likes of lower-priced corn and other vegetable oils. The favorite of Mediterranean cooking often sat ignored on the supermarket shelf because it had a reputation for being too heavy, in taste as well as price. Today, olive oil is the darling of the dining room and the best-loved fat since St. Nick's—all because it's loaded with heart-helping monounsaturated fats.

Monounsaturated fats are thought to protect against heart disease by reducing levels of "bad" LDL cholesterol. But unlike polyunsaturated fats, they may do it without lowering levels of HDL, the "good" cholesterol that we need.

But olive oil's heart-helping qualities don't end there: Researchers from the Lipid Clinic of the Hadassah Hospital in Jerusalem reported that its high percentage of monos may help protect against atherosclerosis by keeping dietary cholesterol and fats from oxidizing. (Oxidation is the chemical process that hardens them into artery-clogging plaque.)

food label, there's a way you can satisfy your curiosity. "Look for the total amount of fat grams, which is listed on many food labels," says Dr. Holub. "Then subtract the grams of saturated fats, polyunsaturated fats and monounsaturated fats. What you have left is trans-fatty acids."

For example, if a product lists seven grams of total fat, three grams of saturated fat, one gram of polyunsaturated and two grams of monounsaturated fat, you would subtract six grams from seven grams. The balance, one gram, is the amount of trans-fatty acids in the product. But some products include trans-fatty acids under monounsaturated fats without making any distinction, which can limit the accuracy of this calculation. To follow Dr. Holub's advice—"the less, the better"—here are some ways to avoid the most obvious sources of trans-fatty acids.

Stand tall against shortening. "A product that boasts 100 percent vegetable shortening may sound healthy, but it's very high in trans-fatty acids," says Litin.

Go soft. Margarine is another unsuspected but major offender, adds Litin. But soft margarine—the kind you buy in tubs—has about one-third the trans-fatty acids of stick margarine.

Say 'bye to fried. Not long ago, many fast-food restaurants switched from frying foods in saturated fats like beef tallow and tropical oils to using "healthier" 100 percent vegetable shortening. Naturally, most people assumed that their french fries and other deep-fried delights were much more heart-healthy than before.

"However," says Litin, "these commercial food products contain 25 to 30 percent trans-fatty acids."

Actually, the hydrogenated vegetable shortenings and oils used now may be as

CARDIO-NUTRIENTS—HEARTTHROB OF THE HEALTHY

The right diet may be one of your best hedges against heart attack. But "right" doesn't end with eating foods that are low in fat, cholesterol and trans-fatty acids. You should also learn to love foods that are high in certain vitamins and minerals that have been found to protect against heart disease. The following are among the most important.

Bolster your betas. Along with fellow "antioxidant" vitamins C and E, beta-carotene protects against heart attack by keeping the harmful form of cholesterol from attaching to artery walls, where it can harden and cause atherosclerosis. The benefits of beta-carotene were discovered in the Physicians Health Study at Harvard Medical School. Results from the research suggested that people who ate the most beta-carotene were only one-fourth as likely to have a heart attack as those who ate the least. Good sources of beta-carotene include sweet potatoes, mangoes, apricots, yellow squash, spinach and broccoli.

Protect yourself with C. Besides keeping plaque from hardening (or "oxidizing"), vitamin C has other benefits. "It can lower the levels of LDL cholesterol while increasing HDL (good cholesterol)," says Aleksandra Niedzwiecki, Ph.D., head of cardiovascular research at the Linus Pauling Institute of Science and Medicine in Palo Alto, California.

"Vitamin C also helps to keep artery walls healthy," she says. Some of the best sources are orange juice, cantaloupe, broccoli, brussels sprouts, green peppers, strawberries and kiwi fruit.

Increase your E. Of the three antioxidant vitamins, the big E has the best antioxidizing effect. In fact, Harvard researchers say that by taking 100 international units daily, women can cut their risk of heart disease by nearly half and men can reduce it by one-third. One problem: Vitamin E is highest in food sources that should be used sparingly, like cooking oils and margarine. A supplement may be your best route to get the E you need, but also try to eat pumpkin seeds, cashews, Brazil nuts, almonds, sunflower seeds and ready-to-eat cereals.

Multiply magnesium. Eating a high-magnesium diet after a heart attack can slash the postepisode death rate by 55 percent, report the National Institutes of Health. It may also be a good preventive measure, adds Forrest Nielsen, Ph.D., director of the U.S. Department of Agriculture Human Nutrition Research Center in Grand Forks, North Dakota. "A lack of dietary magnesium can lead to irregular heartbeats, and magnesium also may keep cholesterol from oxidizing, much like the antioxidant vitamins," he says. Some of the best food sources include bananas, prunes, apricots and pears.

---

bad or even worse than the animal fats the restaurants were using before, according to Dr. Holub. For instance, it used to be that half the fat in some fast-food fries was saturated and could raise cholesterol levels. Now there may not be as much saturated fat, but if you add the saturated and trans-fats, the total is often greater. Says Dr. Holub: "Fried foods in general, and particularly those served in fast-food restaurants, have the most trans-fats of just about any food." And, he adds, it doesn't matter which fried food you choose—fries, chicken or fish.

Make it yourself. Pancake mixes, ready-to-eat waffles, cookies, cakes and other "prepackaged" foods all contain trans-fats in varying amounts, adds Dr. Holub. You can usually decrease the amount of trans-fats (and saturated fats) by making these foods yourself.

"Just adapt the recipes somewhat and use cooking oils in place of margarine or butter—or use half margarine and half oil," suggests dietitian Lisa Litin.

OIL MIXED UP

Actually, cooking oils may present their own problem. Sure, some cooking oils are among the best food sources of polyunsaturated and monounsaturated fats, which can actually help reduce your risk of heart attack by lowering cholesterol. And they have other benefits as well: Vegetable oils are among the highest food sources of vitamin E, the nutrient considered one of the most important in protecting people against heart disease.

But the news about monos and polys is not entirely good, despite their benefits. The problem is, oils are probably the single biggest source of "hidden" fats in the American diet.

"Many people think they can eat anything they want as long as they add some unsaturated salad oil. But that's not the way it is," says Robert Nicolosi, Ph.D., professor of clinical science and director of cardiovascular research at the University of Massachusetts in Lowell. "You have to have these oils rich in monounsaturated and polyunsaturated fats as a *substitute* for saturated fats. Unfortunately, what a lot of people do is overdo it by adding more mono- or polyunsaturated oils, thinking they're doing themselves a favor."

All cooking oils pack a lot of calories in a little bit—120 per tablespoon. And we tend to go overboard with cooking oil. Some people use several tablespoons of oil to coat a 12-inch frying pan when one to two teaspoons will do.

For the same reason you'd avoid these oils on a weight-loss program, you also need to avoid them for the sake of your heart. The extra pounds added to your girth can increase the risk of heart attack as much as monounsaturated or polyunsaturated fats can lower that risk. But here's how to convert your oil consumption, no matter how healthy your choice of oil.

Stir-fry with orange juice. "One of the things we do at my house to reduce the risk of heart attack is to stir-fry a lot of meals," says Dr. Nicolosi. "The key, however, is to use as little oil as possible—ideally, no more than one tablespoon of oil, and preferably just a few drops. You replace the rest of the oil with orange juice, which works very well and adds a great flavor to whatever you're cooking."

Brush, don't pour. Instead of pouring cooking oil into a pan, apply about one teaspoon with a small pastry brush or rub it on with a paper towel. When you use this method to prevent food from sticking, you'll be adding a lot less oil. That alone can cut several hundred calories from a meal.

Use a fraction of what the recipe suggests. In most cases, you can use half the oil called for in a recipe without af-fecting the way the dish tastes. In recipes that specifically call for very flavorful (and saturated) fats, use no more than one-quarter of the suggested amount and make up the difference with one-quarter unsaturated vegetable oil. Then mix that oil duo half-and-half with water, vinegar or stock.

Don't assume light is right. The calorie content is the same in light olive oil as in other oils. The *light* refers to a milder flavor, which results from the way the oil is processed.

WHEN GOOD FOODS TURN BAD

Oils aren't the only reputed heart-healthy foods that have hidden fat. In fact, our diet is full of sneaky fat contributors, which probably explains why, in this era of lean eating, we're consuming more calories than ever before.

Since the 1980s, hundreds of low-fat products have been introduced to help people overcome their heart-hurting eating habits and reduce or reverse their risk of heart attack. And while most Americans believe they practice what is preached, a survey of the eating habits of 15,000 Americans by the National Center for Health Statistics suggests another conclusion.

In the past decade, the survey found, the typical American's intake of saturated fats fell a mere 1 percent, from 13 percent to 12 percent of calories. Americans are still eating as many as 60 more fat calories per day than they should—which is about 2 or 3 percent more saturated fat calories than the AHA recommends. And that recommendation is just to lower the chance of a heart attack, not reverse the risk. To actually reverse the risk, we would probably have to cut down to about half our current level of saturated fats, according to Dr. Stone of Northwestern University School of Medicine.

The reason for our snail-like progress may be partly due to the very foods we consider our salvation. Despite their claims of being cholesterol-free and low in saturated fat, many of these items are

WHAT TO EAT AFTER A HEART ATTACK

Eating plenty of fiber may be the key to recovering from a heart attack. A study from India found that, following a heart attack, patients who ate a low-fat diet that included 52 grams of fiber each day—about twice the amount most Americans eat—had significantly fewer complications and a quicker recovery than those who ate just low-fat foods.

Most of the added fiber came from fruits and vegetables high in antioxidant vitamins C and E and beta-carotene.

To speed their recovery, the patients also had twice as many food sources rich in magnesium. The bounce-back stars also ate one-third less meat and other animal foods than people in the other group—even though total calorie consumption was similar.

loaded with unsuspected trans-fats that increase the "bad" (LDL) cholesterol, lower the "good" (HDL) cholesterol and increase the risk of heart attack. These foods are often high in total fat, which contributes to obesity and heart disease. In addition to the fat-cutting tactics you use to lose weight (see page 44), you can take some additional measures that will also help reduce your risk of heart attack. In the high hidden-fat department, here are some of the worst offenders since the recent charge of the "Lite" Brigade.

Reconsider that morning muffin. You may think you're choosing a low-fat breakfast, but most ready-made muffins sold at supermarkets and coffee shops often have more fat than a similar-size doughnut, because they're loaded with cooking oils. In addition, a store-bought muffin may be merely masquerading as healthful, since many are high in trans-fatty acids, adds Canadian nutrition researcher Dr. Holub.

Here's one way to tell if your muffin is high in fat. Leave the muffin on a paper napkin for about ten minutes. If there's a spot on the napkin when you remove the muffin, rub it to find out if it's greasy. A grease spot means your muffin is full of fat and probably not a health bargain.

Give a cold shoulder to frozen foods. Processed foods, TV dinners and other frozen foods tend to be very high in fat— even if they claim to be otherwise, according to nutritionists. The manufacturers add more fat than you'd find in a similar meal that you'd prepare yourself, because fat gives food more flavor.

The bottom line is that some frozen

FISHING FOR FLAVOR

With so many choices available, it's easy to be left in a sea of confusion. But here's what to look for in tasty fish.

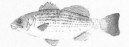

Bass. The meat tastes sweet, but most cooks recommend that you remove the skin before cooking. Otherwise, the flavor of this fish may be a little "off."

Mackerel. The best time to buy is May to July. This relatively oily fish can use a tart-tasting accompaniment like lemon, tomatoes and dry wine.

Get Hooked

Flavorful fish has about one-third the fat of an equal portion of beef. The omega-3 fatty acids in many fish help lower the liver's production of VLDL (very-low-density lipoprotein), a bad type of blood fat, and raise HDL, the good cholesterol linked to heart attack protection. Omega-3's also may reduce the likelihood of blood clots—a leading cause of heart attack. If you're shopping for fish, check the table below for some of the top sources of omega-3's. Also keep in mind the following freshness tips.

Seafood (3 oz.)	Omega-3's (g.)
Anchovies, canned in olive oil	1.8
Atlantic herring	1.8
Pink salmon, canned	1.5
Atlantic sardines, canned	1.3
Bluefin tuna	1.3
Atlantic mackerel	1.1
Sockeye salmon	1.1
Bluefish	0.8
Rainbow trout	0.8
Swordfish	0.8
Albacore tuna, canned in water	0.7
Freshwater bass	0.7
Sea bass	0.7
Pompano	0.6
Halibut	0.5
Chinook salmon (lox), smoked	0.4
Flounder	0.2

Eyes: Look for eyeballs that are clear, bright and bulging. Slightly milky eyeballs mean freshness is fading; sunken, opaque, white or gray eyes mean the fish is bad news.

Gills: Look for a bright red, almost burgundy color that's moist and glistening. Pink gills are okay. Pass on any fish with gray or brown gills with slime. (Incidentally, have the gills removed if you intend to cook the whole fish.)

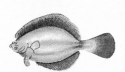

Flounder. Look for fillets with bluish-gray flesh; a milky surface means it's been dipped in preserving solution.

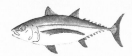

Tuna. This fish is best when barbecued. Slice steaks one inch thick and brush lightly with olive oil. Grill 10 to 12 minutes.

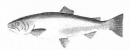

Salmon. The front loin of fillets is tastiest. Remove the skin for soups or casseroles; otherwise leave intact.

dinners have twice as much fat as the same dish you'd prepare yourself. Most are also very high in sodium.

Example: A six-ounce serving of frozen pasta primavera has 305 calories and over 14 grams of fat, and it gets nearly half its calories from fat. It also has 1,410 milligrams of sodium—the entire daily requirement for some people. Make it yourself, though, using the same pasta and vegetables (but fewer of the other fatty and salty ingredients) and a six-ounce portion has only 267 calories, 7 grams of fat and 220 milligrams of sodium.

Don't chicken out at fast-food joints. A typical fast-food meal of a burger, fries and a chocolate milkshake contains almost as much fat as some people should have in an entire day. But if you're looking for a lower-fat alterna-

Skin and flesh: Skin should be bright, shiny and smooth, with tight scales. Loose, dried scales indicate an old fish. Press down to test the flesh. It should be firm and spring back. If a dent remains, freshness is a memory.

Odor: The nose knows—so start at the gut cavity. Off-odors start there. Remember, all fish smell like fish, but a "clean" smell indicates freshness.

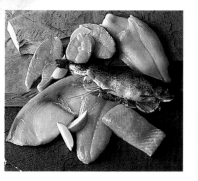

Cuts of fish: Ready for cooking (clockwise from the top)— salmon tail steak, boned flounder fillet, salmon tail and loin fillets, double swordfish steak and salmon steak. A butterflied trout is in the center.

tive, don't assume that chicken is automatically a much better choice. Any fast-food chicken that's dipped in batter and fried is loaded with fat. But if you order a grilled chicken sandwich, you get less fat and fewer calories.

Become a bar attender. Salad bar, that is. You're on the right track if you belly up to the salad bar—instead of ordering from the menu—at your local restaurant or favored fast-food hangout.

But be sure to scoop up the leafy green vegetables, cucumbers, tomatoes, carrots and broccoli. And avoid toppings like cheese, ham, full-fat dressing and creamy goodies like macaroni salad or potato salad. Otherwise, you're getting even more fat than you'd get in a burger. If you make the mistake of ordering a fully loaded taco salad in the shell, you're looking at 60 grams of total fat, the same amount you'd get in four cheeseburgers!

EAT LIKE A EUROPEAN

Of course, the *way* you eat also makes a difference. And if you don't believe it, just look at the other side of the Atlantic. The French, for instance, practically live on cheese, butter and other foods that are rich in saturated fats, but France still has a very low rate of heart disease.

Medical researchers call this the French Paradox. It's been puzzled over since the 1950s, when researchers first noticed that countries whose populations had the most fat in their diets tended to have the highest rates of heart disease—and then noticed that France was a glaring exception.

Several explanations were offered. First, the French traditionally drink a lot of wine, which some experts say helps raise artery-scouring HDL cholesterol. Second, they tend to consume more vegetables and less meat. But still, the average Parisian eats more fat and cholesterol than the average Philadelphian—yet we Americans have twice the rate of heart attack. And many other European countries have the same low rate of death from heart disease as France, although they do not share the same diet.

Researchers then considered the *way* they eat. "It's not just the American diet that's bad, but also our eating habits," says University of Massachusetts nutrition expert Dr. Nicolosi. "Besides reducing the saturated fats and dietary cholesterol in your diet, the way to a lower the risk of heart attack, I believe, is to exercise more and practice eating habits more like the Europeans'." Here's how to do it.

Don't watch the clock. "Our first mistake," explains Dr. Nicolosi, "is that we usually eat on cue. When the clock says it's 8:00 or 9:00 A.M., we have to have breakfast. When it strikes noon, we have to have lunch. We may be eating those meals more out of habit than hunger. When you do that, you tend to eat more throughout the day than you should."

Eat more, early. "Here in the United States, a typical dinner can be at least 1,500 calories—and that's way too much for late in the day," says Dr. Nicolosi. "Compare that to France and other countries, where most of the day's calories are consumed at breakfast and lunch. That gives people plenty of time to burn off their calories." By having your bigger meals earlier in the day, you'll be more likely to lose weight, because eating a lot just before you're ready turn in for the night is one sure way to contribute to obesity.

Desert your favorite dessert. Sweet-

ONION: A FOOD TO BEAT HEART ATTACK

Next time you order a burger, don't hold the onion. The sulfur compounds in onions that make your eyes water also help raise the "good" HDL cholesterol that helps clean artery walls, says nutritional counselor Dr. Isabella Lipinska.

Onions also help decrease triglycerides and may also have a "thinning" effect on the blood that lessens the risk of blood clots. But what's most exciting about onions is that they may actually make fatty meals less dangerous.

"After you have a fatty meal, there is an influx of fat entering your bloodstream, which can raise your risk of heart attack," says Dr. Lipinska. "Onions help prevent this influx of fat because of the sulfur compounds, so if you have onions with that fatty meal, you'll lessen its negative effects."

It takes only about one medium onion a day to get these benefits. And to make onions even more healthy, you can "sweat" them so they'll cook fat-free.

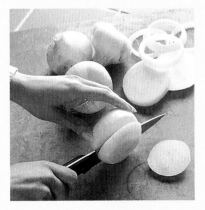

1. To prepare large white onions for "sweating," first cut them into thick slices. Separate the rings.

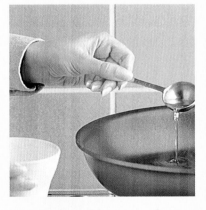

2. Add two tablespoons of chicken broth to a large no-stick skillet. Set on low to medium heat.

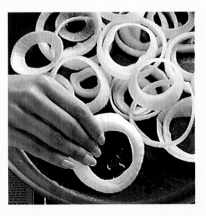

3. Scatter the onion rings in the skillet. Cover tightly with a lid and let the onions "sweat" for about ten minutes.

TAKING GARLIC TO HEART— WITH PILLS

Garlic keeps more away than just vampires: It helps lower cholesterol and "thins" the blood to keep heart attack at bay. Some research shows it may also lower high blood pressure. "Based on our studies, allicin, a constituent of garlic, can decrease the ability of blood to coagulate and can decrease blood pressure in laboratory animals," says Dennis McNamara, Ph.D., of the Department of Pharmacology at Tulane University School of Medicine in New Orleans.

But doctors say you'd have to eat a lot of raw garlic to get these benefits. The alternative is to take garlic tablets. Sold in most drugstores and health food stores, the tablets may give you the benefits of raw garlic, but without heartburn or bad breath.

Look for tablets containing alliin, a precursor of allicin, the active compound believed to produce garlic's heart-helping benefits.

toothed Americans love rich desserts, but overindulging can boost weight and blood cholesterol. If you make the switch to a Mediterranean-style dessert—fruit or low-fat yogurt—you'll trim fat and cholesterol from your diet.

Eat smaller portions. While some Europeans have plenty of fat-filled foods, many—like the French, Italians and Spaniards—just plain eat less. "They eat smaller meals than we do, which is why they don't have the obesity problem—and rate of heart attack," says Dr. Nicolosi.

SMALL CHANGES BRING BIG RESULTS

One of the most effective ways to go beyond holding the line and actually reverse the risk of heart attack is with a regimen prescribed by Dean Ornish, M.D., director of the Preventive Medicine Research Institute in Sausalito, California, and author of *Dr. Dean Ornish's Program for Reversing Heart Disease* and other books. His patients have reversed significant coronary blockages in just one year.

But his program is also one of the toughest: Along with lifestyle changes that include daily stress management and yoga, the program includes a dietary regimen that allows no caffeine, oils or animal products. The only exceptions are dairy products such as low-fat yogurt, nonfat milk and egg whites.

Someone on Dr. Ornish's program gets less than 10 percent of calories from *all* fat sources and almost no cholesterol—as opposed to the maximum of 30 percent of calories from fat and 300 milligrams of cholesterol recommended by the AHA.

But you don't have to go to Ornish-like extremes to see some improvement. Any change for the better is a step in the right direction. Here are some other strategies that can help you reduce your risk.

Go skinless. If you remove the skin of chicken or turkey before you eat it, and you'll avoid 71 percent of its fat

content. It's fine to cook the bird with the skin on, since the fat doesn't "seep" into the meat, but going skinless can slash 50 grams of fat off a typical four-pound chicken.

Don't depend on decaf. Caffeine stresses your heart by making it pump faster, and it also raises triglycerides, a form of fat in the blood that increases risk of heart attack. So many experts advise that those with heart disease should avoid drinking coffee and other beverages that contain caffeine.

But don't depend on decaf to take their place. The oils in decaffeinated coffee actually raise LDL levels more than regular brew, says David Jenkins, M.D., Ph.D., director of the Clinical Nutrition and Risk Factor Modification Center at St. Michael's Hospital at the University of Toronto.

Have an apple a day. Apples contain antioxidant compounds called flavonoids that damage LDL and prevent it from sticking to artery walls. Flavonoids are found in more than 4,000 different foods (including garlic and onions).

Flavonoid-rich apples, however, get a lion's share of research attention. In a five-year study in the Netherlands, researchers found that people who ate an apple a day along with some other flavonoid-rich foods had one-third the heart attack risk of those who didn't eat these foods.

Get the benefits without the breath. Both onions and garlic also raise good cholesterol while decreasing the amount of triglycerides. But both get a bad rap for bad mouth odor.

You don't have to worry, though, says Isabella Lipinska, Ph.D., who is a nutritional counselor for the Cardiac Rehabilitation Program at St. Elizabeth's Hospital in Boston. "By adding garlic and onion to soups, sauces or other cooked foods, you'll get the benefits without the bad breath, and also without the heartburn they can cause. And cooking them doesn't inhibit their heart-protection qualities."

The Heart-Healthy Kitchen

Good-bye to the big black frying pan, swimming in fat, where Grandpa Gump used to fry farm-style flapjacks in bacon grease. Today's cookware of choice, for anyone who wants to avoid fat and cholesterol, is more likely to be no-stick soapstone rather than a greasy skillet. Your kitchen may already be equipped with everything you need to fry, bake and steam in fat-free, nutrient-saving style—but if not, here are some suggested items for the heart-healthy kitchen. The cook's tools on these pages are recommended by experts in the *Prevention* kitchen.

Knives for trimming fat and cutting vegetables include (left to right) a 3" paring knife, 6" and 8" filleting knives and an 8" French knife or chef's knife.

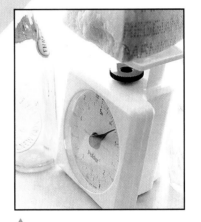

With a food scale, you can weigh food portions before cooking, allowing you to monitor the amount of fat in your diet.

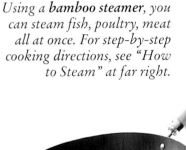

Using a bamboo steamer, you can steam fish, poultry, meat all at once. For step-by-step cooking directions, see "How to Steam" at far right.

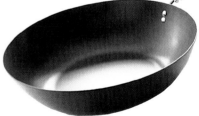

With a no-stick skillet, you can fry or sauté foods with a minimum of oil.

Ribbed, cast-iron fry pans allow the fat to drain off while the meat cooks.

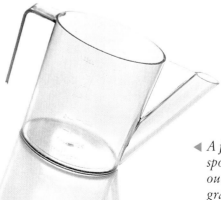

A fat separator has a bottom spout that allows you to pour out fat-free juices for stock and gravy.

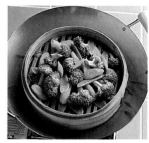

A **stove-top grill topper** allows you to grill meat, fish and vegetables without sautéing in oil.

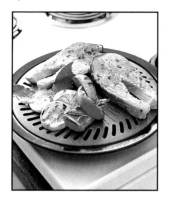

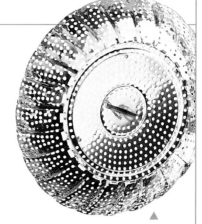

A **stainless steel steamer** holds vegetables above boiling water so they can cook without loss of nutrients.

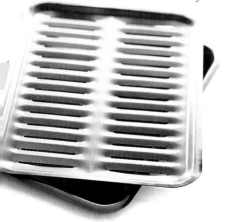

◄ Use a **pastry brush** to apply a very light brushing of oil— minimizing the amount of fat.

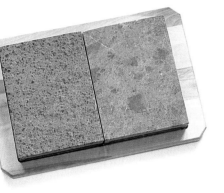

▲ A **soapstone griddle** has a natural nonstick surface, so you don't need cooking oil. The griddle retains heat for a long time.

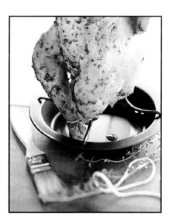

▲ With a **low-fat chicken roaster**, the fat drips into the pan below as the chicken is cooking.

◄ Use a **ladle** as a skimmer to remove unwanted oil or grease from soups and stews.

A **slotted broiler** allows meat juices to drip through to the pan underneath.

1. Place large, chopped vegetables in the steamer bottom. Place it in a wok over an inch or two of boiling water.

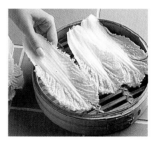

2. To cook fish at the same time, place a layer of bok choy (Chinese cabbage) in the second section of the bamboo steamer.

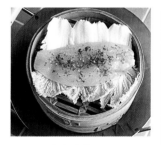

3. Lay fish fillets on top of the bok choy and cover.

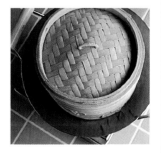

4. Cook for about ten minutes—timing from when the steam first appears.

P A R T
T W O

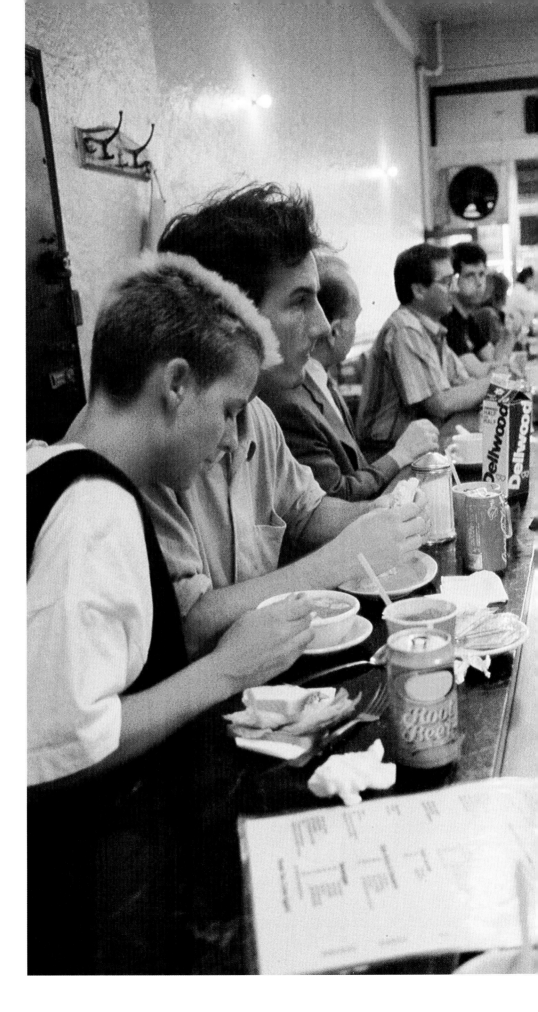

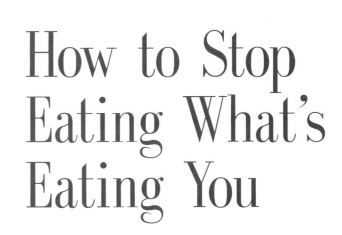

How to Stop Eating What's Eating You

The food

that slims

is the food

that heals

Just a few millennia ago, we humans spent every waking hour mulling over the survival problem—and then doing what had to be done. We farmed, hunted for food, did our short-order cooking over an open fire and dodged the bears, lions and other predators that considered us dessert.

Today, although we're hunting bargains instead of bison and collecting nest eggs instead of duck's eggs, we still have to protect ourselves. Even in today's supermarket, sly saboteurs still lie in wait. Only now they're heavily advertised, and they come disguised in brightly colored packages.

More than 80 million Americans are overweight. This factor alone makes a heavy contribution to our nation's 20 million cases of digestive disorders and 160,000 deaths from diabetes. But it doesn't have to be this way. Whether we're shopping, eating out or stocking the larder, we can detour around the high-fat sections. Choices are important. The foods we select can reduce our glucose to desirable levels, lower a dozen types of risk while also lowering our weight, send surges of nutrients to our healthy cells and tame a bad-tempered intestine.

Whatever the body zone that needs improvement, you can chart your own culinary course for good health. Here's how.

Stop Dieting and Lose Weight: The Proven Way to Lifelong Slimness

You're dying to dig the double fudge chocolate cake out of the bottom of the freezer where you've buried it—beyond reach but not far enough. You think about nuking it in the microwave until it's just barely defrosted, then cutting off slices that melt in your mouth.

But it's bedtime, so you brush your teeth, turn down the sheets and turn out the light. And dream about a life where you could eat without gaining weight, where you wouldn't have to switch to the newest, latest diet every time you need to shed ten pounds.

Dream no more. In fact, you can drive a stake through the word *diet*.

Just switch to low-fat eating. As long as you're eating low-fat foods, "you can eat 'til you feel full," says David Levitsky, Ph.D., professor of nutrition and psychology in the Division of Nutritional Sciences at Cornell University in Ithaca, New York. "And the lower the fat content, the more you can feel free to eat."

One-quarter to one-third of all Americans are overweight, studies say. And 44 million people are dieting at any given time. The average American woman tries at least ten diets in her lifetime, and most of those diets involve some form of calorie restriction.

"Being fat is associated with major medical problems," according to John

WHY FAT'S SO FATTENING

Our bodies make a kind of mincemeat out of the food we eat—breaking it down into grams of fat, protein and carbohydrate. The fat gram is the one to watch out for. The porker of the bunch, it contains nine calories, compared to four calories in each gram of protein or carbohydrate. Also, fat grams are stored in fat cells more efficiently than carbohydrates are. Compare: The body burns just 3 percent of fat calories when it stores the fat we eat in fatty tissue. In the process of storing a carbohydrate in fat tissue, the body burns up 23 percent of calories.

And here's the clincher: The body's fat cells prefer to store fat—so the fat in our diet gets put directly into the fat cells in our body.

At left is a table that will help you limit your fat calories to 25 percent of your daily calorie consumption. First find what your "goal weight" should be and then look for the average number of calories you should get every day. The column at the far right shows the maximum number of calories from fat that should be in your daily diet.

WEIGHT (LB.)	CALORIE INTAKE	FAT LIMIT (G.)
WOMEN		
110	1,300	36
120	1,400	39
130	1,600	44
140	1,700	47
150	1,800	50
160	1,900	53
170	2,000	56
180	2,200	61
Men		
130	1,800	50
140	2,000	56
150	2,100	58
160	2,200	61
170	2,400	67
180	2,500	69
190	2,700	75
200	2,800	78

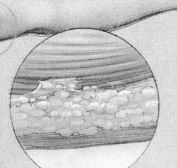

A fat cell is a storage unit that adds bulk to our bodies. A surprisingly dynamic cell, a fat cell is also considered a camel's hump of energy—a buffer against long periods of starvation.

A muscle cell is denser than a fat cell. A combination of low-fat eating and regular exercise will help your body achieve its proper balance of muscle and fat cells.

LOW-FAT FOODS: BUILD MUSCLE CELLS THE EASY WAY

Want to start building muscle? The dinner table may be one ideal place to begin. In fact, low-fat eating may boost lean body mass, or muscle.

This conclusion comes from a study of 18 premenopausal women at the University of Illinois in Chicago. The women went on a low-fat, high-carbohydrate diet that included whole-wheat bread, spaghetti and fruit. After 20 weeks they lost, on average, over 11 percent of their body fat. That was no great surprise.

The 2 percent increase in lean body mass was the kicker. Somehow the women generated new lean tissue without exercise. They didn't have to skimp at the plate, either—they ate more calories in the low-fat phase than in the preceding high-fat phase.

"This is a very intriguing finding," says T. Elaine Prewitt, R.D., Dr.P.H., of the Department of Nutrition at Loyola University Medical Center in Maywood, Illinois. "It may turn out to be a benefit of eating a low-fat diet."

Foreyt, Ph.D., director of the Nutrition Research Clinic at Baylor College of Medicine in Houston and coauthor of *Living without Dieting*. Those problems include heart disease, diabetes and cancer. So if you can get to your ideal weight and stay there, you'll be reducing your health risks in many ways.

WHY DUMP ON DIETS?

It's not that dieters were all the way out in left field when they focused on counting calories. In fact, one of the reasons doctors dislike fat is that a gram of fat has more than twice the calories of a gram of protein or carbohydrate. But if you just focus on reducing the calories in your diet—and don't take steps to specifically eliminate the fat calories—you may skip meals or skimp on portions and end up with a lower-weight body that craves more sustenance or a body with more fat than muscle.

A calorie-free diet of celery and water may help the pounds plummet, but it doesn't help anyone shed weight and keep it off. Hunger only revives ancient caveperson habits, when Adams and Eves binged to store fat in response to famine. "And hunger beats willpower every time. Physiology overcomes psychology," says Dr. Foreyt.

Deprivation diets actually make it harder for you to lose weight. That's because your body regards deprivation as starvation and hangs on to its threatened fat cache for dear life. You wind up burning calories more slowly than you would at normal weight. Your metabolism, the process of turning stored nutrients into energy, actually goes into a slump. For instance, the metabolism of someone on a very low 800-calorie diet can drop by 15 to 20 percent. Essentially, your body compensates for the perceived fuel shortage by slowing

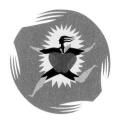

BREAKTHROUGHS IN HEALING

1 9 7 7

Researchers at the University of Vermont in Burlington discover that men on high-fat diets gain weight more than twice as fast as men on mixed fat and carbohydrate diets.

1 9 8 6

Based on research at the University of Pennsylvania School of Medicine in Philadelphia and the National Academy of Sciences in Washington, D.C., doctors advise people who have a family history of obesity to be especially careful about their weight.

1 9 9 1

Researchers studying data from the landmark Framingham Heart Study in Massachusetts find that people whose weight fluctuates often or greatly (yo-yo dieters) have an increased risk of coronary heart disease. They conclude that repeated cycles of drastic dieting, followed by weight gain, are more risky than steady weight gain or permanent weight loss.

down the calorie-burning process.

"Restriction becomes very difficult. You're fighting biology all the way. And it's not nice to try fooling Mother Nature," says Jay Kenney, R.D., Ph.D., nutrition research specialist at the Pritikin Longevity Center in Santa Monica, California.

THE YO-YO: WORSE THAN NO-NO

Experience and research both show that low-calorie, mini-portion diets are almost always fated to flop. So the proven failure rate of 95 percent is not surprising. But the "yo-yo" cycle of starving and eating, losing and gaining, is not only doomed to fail, it's dangerous, a team of researchers from Boston University, Yale University and Bryant College in Smithfield, Rhode Island, discovered.

Reviewing 3,000 health records spanning 32 years of the landmark Framingham Heart Study, the team found that people whose weight fluctuated either often or greatly had a 75 percent greater risk of dying from heart disease than those who had fairly stable weight during those years.

It's not that calories don't matter. They do. But the kind of calories they are—whether they're from fat or protein or complex carbohydrates—matters more. Protein calories power our muscle cells. Carbohydrates are what our bodies use to fuel up and go—whether running in marathons or standing in place. Fat calories all too often wind up just where their name implies—in fat cells as fat.

Both the U.S. Surgeon General and leading weight-loss experts have called for us to reduce the fat in our diet. To do that, we first have to figure out what percentage of our calories comes from dietary fat.

Most Americans get more than 35 percent of their calories from fat. The new target, according to weight-loss experts, is 30 percent. Ideally, you can get down to 25 percent of calories from fat.

In addition, weight-loss experts consistently recommend regular exercise, the Sundance Kid that accompanies the Butch Cassidy of low-fat eating. Because the two get more action when riding together, weight loss is really an exercise-and-low-fat-eating duet rather than a diet.

In fact, "we don't use the word *diet*," says Maria Simonson, Sc.D., Ph.D., director of the Health, Weight and Stress Clinic at Johns Hopkins Medical Institutions in Baltimore. "It sends a shiver down people's spines. We say *eatin program*."

DEFANGING DEPRIVATION

Say you want to get started on a low-fat program. How do you begin? "Very slowly and gradually. If you cut back on fat too quickly, you'll feel deprived," says Dr. Foreyt.

"Be the tortoise instead of the hare," suggests George L. Blackburn, M.D., Ph.D., associate professor of surgery at Harvard Medical School and chief of the Nutrition/Metabolism Laboratory at New England Deaconess Hospital in Boston. "Allow a minimum of 13 to 26 weeks to start eating low-fat—one or two semesters."

Dr. Blackburn warns that it doesn't make sense to cut out all our "comfort foods" the first day or first week of a weight-loss program. In fact, a too-radical change in diet is an invitation to failure, in his view.

First, the experts suggest, take inventory and draw up some lists.

Write in your "Dear Food" diary. Many weight-loss experts suggest keeping a food diary for a few days. List what you ate immediately after you've had a meal or snack.

Noting snacks is important. One of the things you're looking for in your food diary is "hidden fats," says Dr. Foreyt—the peanuts on the airplane or the nighttime glass of whole milk.

Once you've recorded how much food you've eaten for a few days, you can figure out what items you would be most comfortable deleting from your menu, says Ronette Kolotkin, Ph.D., director of Behavioral Programs at the Duke University Diet and Fitness Center in Durham, North Carolina.

Figure your fat budget. Using the table on page 44, find your target weight, ideal calorie intake and fat limit. The fat limit is the maximum number of fat grams that you can have each day. Ideally, that should be no more than 25 percent of your calorie intake. By reading food labels, you can run a daily tab on fat grams, tracking the total from breakfast to bedtime.

Read labels—carefully. Even with newer, easier-to-understand food labels, a quick glance won't give you the real story about a product's fat content. That's because the most important number listed—the percentage of calories that come from fat—aren't for that serving size, as you may think, but for your entire daily allowance.

A case in point: The label of a "low-calorie" salad dressing lists its 5 grams of fat per serving as representing only 8 percent of calories. But unless you read the label carefully, you may not realize that 8 percent is for your entire day's fat "quota," based on a 2,000-calorie intake—and not the mere two-tablespoon serving size.

Also, if a label says "nonfat," it just means that the food has less than one gram of fat per serving. Since most people use more than the suggested serving size, so this fat adds up quickly.

Fatproof your domicile. The Duke University Diet and Fitness Center actually runs a class on fatproofing the kitchen, but here's the basic homework: Go through your kitchen cabinets, remove temptations and make space for some healthy new groceries.

The reason for a reduced-fat household is simple: If you don't have chocolate chip cookies in the cookie jar, you can't eat them.

Plan to personalize. For a reliable weight-loss program, you have to make snacks and meals from foods you really like, says Cheryl Clifford Marco, R.D., dietitian at the Outpatient Nutrition Service of Thomas Jefferson University Hospital in Philadelphia. She believes that liking what you eat can make the difference in losing weight and in keeping it off after you lose it.

Weight-loss experts encourage people to develop a program that makes low-fat eating and exercise more enjoyable. If you develop a plan that includes attitude adjustment, a physical activity program—and all the low-fat foods you like to eat—you'll be more likely to lose weight and keep it off.

SHARP SHOPPING

Before you begin low-fat eating, you have to shop for low-fat food. This

(continued on page 52)

SWAP WHAT'S ON TOP

Have your fill of low-fat food, say weight-loss experts—but be careful you don't sabotage it with what you put on top. Cooked oatmeal, for instance, is a healthy, filling source of fiber. But if you put ½ cup of Half-and-Half and two teaspoons of margarine on it, it becomes 58 percent fat. To scalp the fat, just leave off the margarine and replace the cream with skim milk. Presto—your morning oatmeal is no more than 12 percent fat.

A four-ounce breakfast bagel topped with an ounce of cream cheese is 27 percent fat. Use nonfat cream cheese, though, and the fat content plummets to 8 percent.

If cereal is your breakfast of choice, you can slash fat 28 percent by replacing a cup of whole milk with skim milk—even when you add a banana. If you prefer 2 percent milk to skim, you'll still cut your fat by 18 percent—and that's with the banana, too.

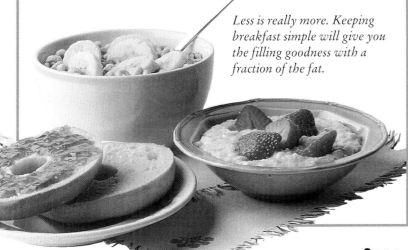

Less is really more. Keeping breakfast simple will give you the filling goodness with a fraction of the fat.

Send in the Substitutes

You can replace almost any high-fat food with its slimmer sister. Here are some ways.

Stir-fry a Polynesian duet. Substitute pineapple juice for oil, then "sauté" broccoli and cauliflower florets.

Sizzle veggies in their own juices. You can "fry" vegetables in their own juices if they have a high moisture content. Place a no-stick pan over low heat, add vegetables and cover. Cook the vegetables until softened, stirring them occasionally.

Decream your coffee. Many people use a nondairy creamer like Cremora, which is 58 percent fat. A simple alternative is to switch to nonfat dry milk powder that has zero fat.

Cut Half-and-Half to zero. Use evaporated skim milk, which is nearly fat-free, instead of Half-and-Half, which is 79 percent fat.

Free your soup. Instead of using heavy cream for a bisque soup, substitute buttermilk (which is equal to 1 percent low-fat milk) or evaporated skim milk.

Researchers have long known that people adapt to low-fat eating better when they use low-fat substitutes in their favorite dishes than when they give up their accustomed fare cold turkey. Here's a table to help you modify the high-fat foods of yesterday into the low-fat—and delicious—favorites of today.

SPEEDY SUBSTITUTIONS	
TO REPLACE	**USE**
1 Tbsp. butter (as a topping)	Salsa, nonfat sour cream, lemon juice, butter-flavored (nonfat) sprinkles
1 cup heavy cream	1 cup evaporated skim milk
1 medium whole egg	¼ cup fat-free egg substitute
1 cup regular yogurt	1 cup nonfat yogurt
1 cup sour cream	1 cup light sour cream or 1 cup nonfat yogurt
1 oz. baking chocolate	3 Tbsp. cocoa powder

HEALTHY HOME COOKING

Don't tear up your favorite family recipes just because they're full of butter or cheese. A low-fat food product or a fat-reducing cooking technique can transform your old standbys.

Apple Pie with Crumb Topping

Removing the traditional crust accounts for the big difference in calories and fat between this apple-crisp-type pie and a standard one.

- 5 medium apples, peeled, quartered and thinly sliced
- ⅓ cup honey
- 1 tablespoon lemon juice
- ¼ cup unbleached flour
- ¼ cup packed light brown sugar
- ¼ teaspoon ground cinnamon
- ¼ teaspoon grated nutmeg
- 2 tablespoons reduced-calorie margarine

In a large bowl, mix the apples, honey and lemon juice. Spoon into a 9" pie plate, mounding the apples in the center.

Place the flour, sugar, cinnamon and nutmeg in a food processor. Process briefly to combine. Cut the margarine into small pieces and distribute on top of the flour mixture. Process with on/off turns until the mixture resembles coarse crumbs.

Sprinkle the crumbs over the apples and pat them into place. Bake at 375° for 45 minutes, or until the apples have softened and the crumbs have browned. Serve with nonfat yogurt topping.

Makes 6 servings.

Per serving (original): *370 calories, 21 g. fat (51% of calories), 2 g. dietary fiber, 27 mg. cholesterol, 259 mg. sodium.* Per serving (low-fat version): *193 calories, 3 g. fat (12% of calories), 2.2 g. dietary fiber, 0 mg. cholesterol, 25 mg. sodium.*

Macaroni and Cheese

Most recipes for macaroni and cheese start with a fatty cream sauce. Our version replaces the sauce with smoothly blended low-fat cottage cheese.

- 1 container (16 ounces) low-fat cottage cheese
- 2 tablespoons skim milk
- 1 tablespoon Dijon mustard
- ½ teaspoon onion powder
- ½ teaspoon ground black pepper
- 8 ounces elbow macaroni
- ¼ cup grated Parmesan cheese
- 2 tablespoons minced fresh parsley

Place the cottage cheese, milk, mustard, onion powder and pepper in a food processor. Process for

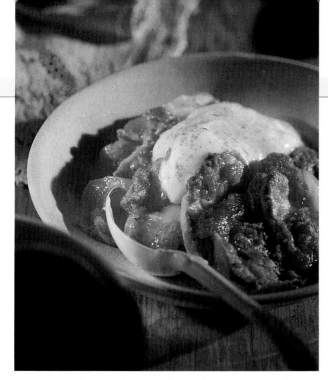

Removing the crust from traditional apple pie transforms it into a low-fat treat.

3 minutes, or until very smooth. Transfer to a 2-quart saucepan. Place over low heat and let warm, stirring often, while the macaroni cooks.

Cook the marcaroni in a large pot of boiling water for 8 minutes, or until tender. Drain and return to the pot. Off heat, add the sauce, mix well, sprinkle with Parmesan and parsley, and toss lightly.

Makes 4 servings.

Per serving (original): *583 calories, 34 g. fat (53% of calories), 0.6 g. dietary fiber, 97 mg. cholesterol, 1,066 mg. sodium.*
Per serving (low-fat version): *329 calories, 4 g. fat (12% of calories), 1 g. dietary fiber, 10 mg. cholesterol, 652 mg. sodium.*

Breaded Chicken

Deep-frying breaded chicken pieces adds a tremendous amount of fat to what's essentially lean meat. Baking the chicken, and removing the skin before breading, produces the same crispy texture without the extra fat.

- 4 skinless, boneless chicken breasts (about 4 ounces each)
- 2 tablespoons all-purpose flour
- ⅓ cup fat-free egg substitute
- ½ cup seasoned dry bread crumbs

Dip the chicken in the flour to coat both sides; shake off any excess.

Place the egg substitute in a shallow bowl and dip the chicken into them to coat both sides.

Place the bread crumbs on a large plate and dip the chicken into them to coat both sides.

Coat a baking sheet with no-stick spray. Place the chicken on the baking sheet in a single layer. Bake at 375° for 25 minutes, or until the pieces are tender and no longer pink in the center.

Makes 4 servings.

Per serving (original): *384 calories, 21 g. fat (50% of calories), 0.6 g. dietary fiber, 113 mg. cholesterol, 209 mg. sodium.*
Per serving (low-fat version): *195 calories, 2 g. fat (10% of calories), 0.6 g. dietary fiber, 66 mg. cholesterol, 192 mg. sodium.*

Meat Loaf

Artful substitution of extra-lean beef and turkey breast slashes fat from this family favorite.

- ¾ cup diced carrots
- ¾ cup diced onions
- ½ cup diced red peppers
- 8 ounces extra-lean ground beef (92% lean)
- 8 ounces ground turkey breast
- 1 cup rolled oats
- ¾ cup tomato juice
- ¼ cup fat-free egg substitute
- 1 teaspoon dried thyme
- ½ teaspoon ground black pepper
- 2 tablespoons ketchup

Coat a large no-stick frying pan with no-stick spray. Add the carrots, onions and red peppers. Sauté for 5 minutes, or until the vegetables are tender; if necessary, add a little water to the pan to keep the vegetables from sticking. Transfer to a large bowl.

Crumble the beef and turkey into the bowl. Add the oats and toss lightly.

In a small bowl, combine the tomato juice, egg substitute, thyme and black pepper. Drizzle over the meat and mix lightly but thoroughly.

Coat an 8½" × 4½" loaf pan with no-stick spray. Transfer the meat mixture to the pan. Spread the ketchup on top.

Bake at 350° for 45 to 50 minutes, or until cooked through. If the top begins to brown too much, cover with a piece of foil. Let stand for about 10 minutes before serving

Makes 4 servings.

Per serving (original): *407 calories, 28 g. fat (64% of calories), 0.4 g. dietary fiber, 112 mg. cholesterol, 695 mg. sodium.*
Per serving (low-fat version): *263 calories, 5 g. fat (19% of calories), 2.8 g. dietary fiber, 67 mg. cholesterol, 158 mg. sodium.*

Lite, Lite-er, Lite-est

Today, there are thousands of low-fat or nonfat foods on supermarket shelves. With so many choices, it's easy to create delicious meals and snacks that contain less than 25 percent of calories from fat. The first column below shows a reasonable and relatively healthy menu for a day of eating. Still, it adds up to 36 percent of calories from fat. But look what happens when you follow the same menu but substitute light versions of the same foods. As you can see, just a few small changes can make a huge difference.

HOW TO DEFAT YOUR MEALS

"BEFORE LIGHT" MENU	PORTION	CALORIES	FAT (G.)	"LIGHT" MENU	PORTION	CALORIES	FAT (G.)	"IDEAL" MENU	PORTION	CALORIES	FAT (G.)
BREAKFAST				**BREAKFAST**				**BREAKFAST**			
Cranberry juice	4 oz.	72	<1	Orange-cranberry juice	4 oz.	63	<1	Cranberry juice	4 oz.	72	<1
Bagel	1	163	1	Bagel	1	163	1	Oatmeal, cooked	1/2 cup	104	2
Cream cheese	1 oz.	100	10	Cream cheese, light	1 oz.	74	7	Blueberries, fresh	1 cup	41	<1
Fruit-flavored yogurt, low-fat	8 oz.	231	2 1/2	Yogurt, light	8 oz.	107	<1	Plain yogurt, nonfat	1 cup	127	<1
LUNCH				**LUNCH**				**LUNCH**			
Sandwich:				Sandwich:				Sandwich:			
Whole-wheat bread	2 slices	131	2	Whole-wheat bread	2 slices	131	2	Whole-wheat bread	2 slices	131	2
Ham, low-sodium, 96% fat-free, cooked	1 oz.	30	1	Ham, 96% fat-free	1 oz.	30	1	Tuna salad	3 oz.	100	2
Mozzarella cheese, skim	1 oz.	72	4 1/2	Mozzarella cheese, skim	1 oz.	72	4 1/2	Mayonnaise, light, low-cal	1 tsp.	40	4
Mayonnaise	1 Tbsp.	100	11	Mayonnaise, low-fat, low-cal	1 Tbsp.	40	4	Alfalfa sprouts	1/4 cup	3	<1
Romaine lettuce	1/4 cup	2	<1	Romaine lettuce	1/4 cup	2	<1	Romaine lettuce	1/4 cup	2	<1
Tomato	1/2	13	<1	Tomato	1/2	13	<1	Tomato	1/2	13	<1
Minestrone soup	1/2 cup	41	1	Minestrone soup	1/2 cup	41	1	Black turtle bean soup	1/2 cup	109	<1
Apple	1	81	<1	Apple	1	81	<1	Apple	1	81	<1
SNACK				**SNACK**				**SNACK**			
Microwave popcorn	3 cups	210	13	Microwave popcorn, light	3 cups	70	3	Hot-air-popped popcorn with chili powder	3 cups	75	0
DINNER				**DINNER**				**DINNER**			
Tossed salad	1 cup	32	<1	Tossed salad	1 cup	32	<1	Tossed salad	1 cup	16	<1
Italian dressing	2 Tbsp.	137	14	Italian dressing, light	2 Tbsp.	32	3	Italian dressing, reduced-calorie	2 Tbsp.	32	3
Chicken breast, no skin, roasted	3 oz.	140	3	Chicken breast, no skin, roasted	3 oz.	140	3	Vegetable lasagna, frozen, low-fat	1 1/2 cups	390	12
Broccoli, cooked	1/2 cup	12	<1	Broccoli, cooked	1/2 cup	12	<1	Italian bread	2 slices	170	0
Margarine	1 tsp.	34	4	Margarine, light	1 tsp.	21	2	Margarine, light	1 tsp.	21	2
Baked potato	1	145	<1	Baked potato	1	145	<1	Poached pear	1	83	<1
Sour cream	1 Tbsp.	62	6	Sour cream, light	2 Tbsp.	40	6	**SNACK**			
Coffee	1 cup	5	0	Coffee	1 cup	5	0	Frozen yogurt, fruit-flavored	1 cup	216	2
Nondairy creamer	1 Tbsp.	24	0	Half & Half	1 Tbsp.	16	0				
Devil's food cake	1 slice	235	8	Chocolate cake, frozen	1 slice	170	8				
SNACK				**SNACK**							
Vanilla ice cream	1/2 cup	135	7	Vanilla ice cream, light	1/2 cup	92	3				

Total calories: 2,205
Total fat: 90 g.
Percent of calories from fat: 36
Total cholesterol: 229 mg.

Total calories: 1,602
Total fat: 44 g.
Percent of calories from fat: 24
Total cholesterol: 128 mg.

Total calories: 1,847
Total fat: 32 g.
Percent calories from fat: 16
Total cholesterol: 48 mg.

Tasty Delites

Light foods are miracles of chemistry. "Low-fat mayonnaise (to take just one example) is a technological achievement," says Seattle researcher and chef Dr. Alan Kristal. But do the light foods really taste good?

To find the answer, a team of taste testers from *Prevention* magazine raided the food market shelves to find the best of the low-fat and nonfat alternatives. Taste is subjective, of course—so the final test is your own. But here are the products that made the biggest impression on the *Prevention* staff.

Granolas. The old first-generation granolas were crunchingly high in fat—about six grams an ounce, with an average portion being perhaps two or three times that much. Then came low-fat granolas, with just two grams of fat, followed by nonfat varieties. Our tasters tucked into the date-and-almond variety of Health Valley Fat-Free Granola and came away saying, "Nice crunch!"

Pancakes. Aunt Jemima Low-Fat Pancakes have two grams of fat in three pancakes instead of the six grams you'd get in the homemade variety. Reactions: "Hey, pretty good for a pancake you just pop into the toaster!"

Pasta sauce. Typical pasta sauce has about five grams of fat per half cup, so a nonfat version really makes a difference. The *Prevention* staff tried two varieties, and the clear winner was the garlic and onion flavor of Healthy Choice Pasta Sauce. Typical comments: "Excellent . . . nice mix of flavors . . . delicious!"

Munchies. Among the *Prevention* tasters, Nabisco's Snack Well Line proved very popular. They especially liked the Cracked Pepper Crackers and Cinnamon Graham Snacks. And they gave very high ratings to Armsnack Rice Snax (herb and garlic), which have one gram of fat per half-ounce (about 14 pieces).

Among fat-free potato chips, the winner was Louise's Fat-Free Potato Chips, which have a "natural oil flavor" that proved appealing. And the total fat saving was ten grams per ounce.

For a universal thumbs-up from all the tasters, the winner was Guiltless Gourmet Mild Black Bean Dip. Every synonym for "Terrific!" was used to laud the taste of this healthy snack. A fan noted that the spicy version tasted even better than the mild one.

Chocolate pudding. The tasters favored Hunt's Snack Pack Fat-Free Chocolate Pudding, but they also liked Hershey's Free Chocolate Bar Flavor Pudding and Swiss Miss Fat-Free Chocolate Pudding. Each has six grams less fat than regular pudding.

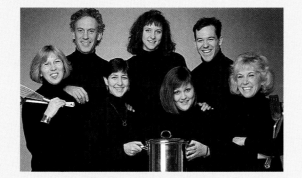

A tough job, but someone has to do it! Editors, writers and researchers from Prevention *magazine eagerly tasted—and evaluated—the best of the low-fat fare.*

A Consumer's Guide to the New Faux Fats

Every week, three out of every four people use a reduced-fat food of some kind. But do we know what replaces the butter and oil?

■ *Most of the fake fats started out somewhere in nature. Those made from carbohydrates appear on labels as dextrin, maltodextrin and modified food starches. Right now, there are about 20 plant-based fat substitutes that began life as wheat, potatoes, corn or rice. They spare us five calories a gram and show up in foods like salad dressings, sauces and low-fat or fat-free mayonnaise. The carbohydrate fat substitutes are stable enough for use in baking but not in frying.*

■ *The best-known phony fat is Simplesse, from the NutraSweet Company. It's made from the protein of egg whites or milk whey. Simplesse has 1⅓ calories per gram instead of fat's 9 calories per gram, and it's used in frozen desserts like frozen yogurt and ice cream. One drawback is in cooking: Simplesse gels at high heat, so you can't bake or fry with it.*

■ *Olestra, another brand of fat substitute, is made from sugar and oil. Like water and some forms of fiber, Olestra provides no additional fat or calories. Its inventor, Procter and Gamble, hopes to use it to replace all the vegetable shortening or oil in salted snacks like potato chips and corn chips. It may also be good for cooking.*

Besides helping you cut fat and calorie consumption, the faux fats try to provide the consistency and texture that real fat gives to so much food. At their best, these substitutes mimic the "mouthfeel" of fat—the long, slow, creamy sensation you get when eating gourmet ice cream, for example.

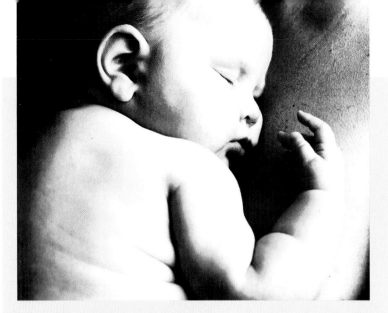

How New Moms Lose

Junior's not the only one who gets benefits from breast-feeding. Studies suggest it can also help Mom ease back into her prepregnancy clothes.

In one study, researchers found that mothers who breast-fed their babies for more than six months lost about ten pounds during the baby's first year, while those using formula lost a little more than five pounds.

The key is to eat what you normally would, according to Kathryn G. Dewey, Ph.D., professor of nutrition at the University of California, Davis. That might be a little tough the first few months, she notes, because the milk-inducing hormone, prolactin, may increase your appetite. But after the first three months, the study suggests, mothers who breast-feed their babies get the weight-loss edge over those using formula.

means you're up against major marketing techniques that are designed to lead you into a superfatted maze. But if you employ some defatting techniques, you can win the skirmishes with advertising.

Scope out labels. "People who are starting to eat low fat should check out food labels," says Liz Applegate, Ph.D., nutrition lecturer at the University of California, Davis, and author of *Power Foods*. The labels on processed foods tell you the amount of fat calories in a serving of the product and the number of fat grams per serving.

Supermarkets don't need to have signs that lead you to low-fat foods. The labels on most canned and packaged foods have fat information to help you out. (Unfortunately, many of the foods imported from other countries do not have labels with the usual nutritional information.) The good news is that there are low-fat foods that don't need labels—they're all in the produce section. Loading up the grocery cart with fruits and vegetables is a sure way to take the fat out of your frying pan.

Breads and the like are starches, but so are fruits and vegetables. All complex carbohydrates are starches made up of long chains of sugar molecules. And they're not fat-builders.

Your body would much rather burn carbohydrates as fuel than attempt to store them as fat. That's because the body has to work to break down the long chains of sugar molecules into simple sugars—only then can it convert a complex carbohydrate into fat. By contrast, dietary fat slips into a fat cell as easily as a housecat sneaks in the back door. So every time you eat complex carbohydrates instead of fat, you're choosing to burn calories rather than store fat.

Never shop on empty. Eat before you shop—and that means for anything, clothes as well as food. Food courts and fast-food restaurants at malls are as tempting as cookie aisles in supermarkets. If you can't eat beforehand or if you're shopping till you drop, take along an apple or banana so you won't run on empty, suggests Debra Waterhouse, R.D., a nutritionist in private practice and author of *Outsmarting the Female Fat Cell*. "Don't let yourself get too hungry," says Waterhouse.

Stay outside. If you don't have time to read the food labels on a given day, stick to the outside aisles of the supermarket. That's where many complex carbohydrates—including fresh fruits, vegetables and bread—reside. The middle aisles are the heart of darkness—a high-fat jungle with labels like exotic orchids.

Nix all nuts but one. Reading food labels will show you that nuts are fraught with fat—from peanuts, which have 14 grams of fat per ounce, to macadamias, with 21 fat grams per ounce. There is one good nut, however. It's the chestnut, which contains about ½ gram of fat per ounce. "We underutilize chestnuts. They have a wonderful flavor," says Ruth Spear, author of *Low Fat and Loving It.*

Maybe one reason we don't eat more chestnuts is because they're a pain to peel. But you can make them easier to peel if you just slit the chestnuts with a knife on the flat side, making an *X* in the shell before you roast them. Then place them on a baking sheet and roast at 425°F for 15 to 20 minutes.

Don't let Ben and Jerry out of the store. Once you've fatproofed your domicile, "you have to plan your shopping so that you keep problem foods out of the house," says Dr. Kolotkin of the Duke University Diet and Fitness Center.

If you have a yearning for premium ice cream, the last thing you need in your freezer is a pint of temptation, weighing in with over 60 percent fat. It's just too easy to scoop out some Chunky Monkey if you bring it home.

"If you really want to have ice cream, cookies or junk food, go ahead and have them—but have them outside the house," suggests Dr. Kolotkin. "Go to the ice cream store and order a scoop of premium ice cream. This way it's in a controlled environment and you can't finish off a pint by yourself."

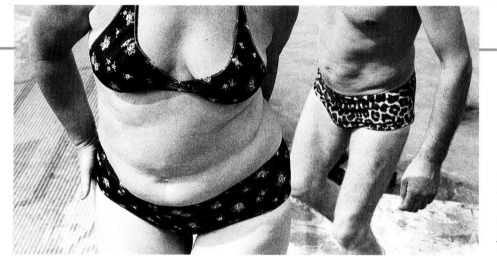

In the quest for perpetual slimness, men have the edge. Research shows their cells give up fat more readily than women's do.

SEXIST FAT CELLS

Fat's not fair. "Men have an easier time with weight loss because their fat cells are smaller to begin with," says nutritionist and dietitian Debra Waterhouse.

Women's fat cells need to be big enough to store extra reserves, and while those reserves are necessary during pregnancy, it may be hard to lose weight when these cells are designed for extra storage. But there's another reason, apart from size, that women's cells are plumper than men's. Women, according to Waterhouse, have more lipogenic enzymes that help store the fat more easily and efficiently. Men, by contrast, have more lipolytic enzymes that help yank fat out of the cells for use elsewhere in the body. The upshot is that men can lose weight faster than women even when they eat the same amount and types of food.

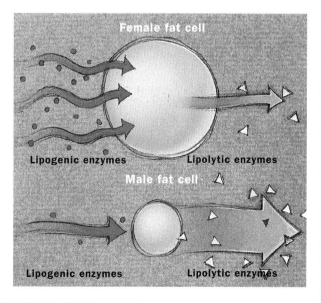

S.O.S. Snacks

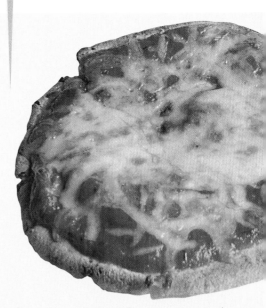

You get home, hang up your coat and head for the kitchen. It's 30 minutes until mealtime, but your stomach feels like a hollow drum. And the drum is starting to boom, "Feed me!"

If you're going to outsmart the urging of your stomach, you'll want to have a medley of low-fat snacks on hand.

In fact, many weight-loss experts recommend more healthy snacking and less large-portion dining. One study even showed that lean women tended to eat four meals a day, or even more than that. So if you're eating by the clock, you're better off eating smaller meals more often. Here are some ideas for guilt-free snacks and mini-meals.

TURKEY TALK

Keep sliced, roast turkey breast in the fridge for sandwiches. (When freshly sliced, it will keep for two to five days.) Then line a pita bread "pocket" with lettuce and tuck in the turkey.

SUNDAE SLIM

Layer nonfat frozen yogurt with chopped fruit and preroasted chestnuts in a sundae dish. Try vanilla with chopped banana or strawberry with sliced strawberries.

PASTA PETITE

Put last night's fresh pasta in a sealed plastic bag in the fridge, tossed with a smidgen of olive oil to keep it from clumping up. (For a new pasta sensation, try tomato rotini or carrot elbows.) Make an instant salad by tossing 1 tablespoon nonfat dressing with 1 cup pasta. Toss in some leftover vegetables, too.

SWEET SANDWICH

Make "ice cream sandwiches" by spreading slightly softened nonfat frozen yogurt between two low-fat oatmeal cookies or graham crackers. Store them, tightly wrapped, in the freezer.

FAST FRUIT

Peel and section citrus fruits. For a quick treat, mix pink grapefruit with oranges and tangerines.

TOP POPS

Popped corn is a great high-fiber snack, and a hot-air popper keeps the

PRONTO PIZZA

For the world's quickest pizza, first split an English muffin or pita.

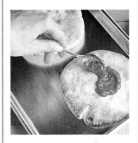

Spread it with a bit of tomato paste and Italian spices.

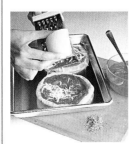

Sprinkle shredded nonfat mozzarella on top and place under the broiler until the cheese has melted.

fat content down. Toss your popped corn with raisins and cooked, chopped chestnuts for more flavor.

QUICK QUENCHER

Keep seltzer water on hand, along with a variety of fruit juices. Then you can create your own healthful sodas. Try ½ cup seltzer, ¼ cup orange juice and ¼ cup purple grape juice.

SKINNY SKINS

For delicious potato-skin snacks, bake extra potatoes and stash them in the fridge. When you're ready, halve the potatoes and scoop out the insides with a spoon, leaving about ¼ inch of flesh. Sprinkle with shredded reduced-fat cheddar cheese and minced chives. Broil about 5½ inches from the heat source until the potatoes are warmed through and the cheese has melted, about four minutes.

BULGELESS WAFFLES

Heat a frozen waffle according to package directions. Top with maple yogurt, made by folding together equal parts of maple syrup and plain nonfat yogurt. Add sliced bananas or apples.

DESIGNER DIP

For an easy and delicious dip, combine ½ cup nonfat ricotta and ½ cup nonfat yogurt. Stir in 1 to 2 teaspoons of your favorite herbs, such as basil, dill and tarragon. Enjoy with slices of fresh vegetables or reduced-fat whole-wheat crackers.

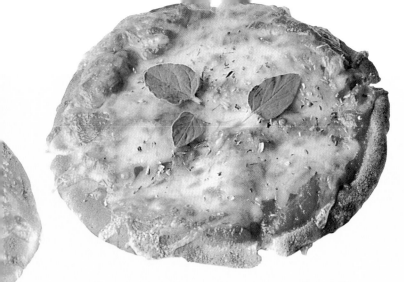

Pronto Pizza

VEGGIES ON THE MOVE

Try some new raw vegetables and keep them in bite-size pieces in the fridge. Eat them either with or without your favorite low-fat dip. Cherry tomatoes, sugar snap peas, cut-up rutabaga, whole white mushrooms, Jerusalem artichokes, cut-up fennel bulb, Chinese cabbage ribs, sliced celeriac, sliced daikons and some jicama chunks can perk up your palate.

PLEASED CHEESE

Nibble on strips of low-fat cheese and strips of sweet red, yellow and green peppers or chunks of carrots.

SVELTE DRESSING

Here's a dressing to keep on hand for a zippy pasta salad. Place ½ cup nonfat cottage cheese, ¼ cup chopped red onions, 1 tablespoon skim milk, a dash of ground cumin and a chopped sprig of dill in a food processor or blender. Process on low to medium speed until very smooth. Refrigerate until chilled.

APPLE DELHI DIP

For a tasty fruit dip, place ½ cup nonfat cottage cheese, ¼ cup apple juice, ½ teaspoon curry powder and a dash each of cinnamon, nutmeg and fresh chopped mint in a blender. Process on low to medium speed until very smooth. Keep chilled in a bowl in the refrigerator.

FISH IN A FLASH

In a blender or food processor, puree 6 tablespoons nonfat cottage cheese, 1 tablespoon Dijon mustard and 1 teaspoon each of dill, parsley and chives. Add 1 cup cubed cooked leftover flounder or other white fish and puree on medium to high speed until combined. Keep it in a crock in the fridge; it makes an excellent spread to go with low-fat whole-grain crackers.

SUMMER FAST FRUIT

Keep chunks of mango and nectarines, along with seedless green grapes and pitted cherries, in plastic bags in the freezer. They're quick refreshers—as good as ice pops.

INSTANT NACHOS

These quick and tasty nachos take less than five minutes to make, and they're great snacks. Keep some soft flour tortillas and light Monterey Jack cheese in the refrigerator and you can create these nachos at the drop of a Mexican hat.

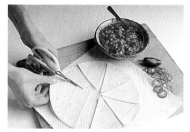

Before putting on toppings, it's a good idea to crisp the tortilla in a microwave. Line a plate with a paper towel. Cut the tortilla into eighths with kitchen shears and arrange the pieces around the plate's rim. Microwave uncovered on full power until just crisp, about 1½ minutes.

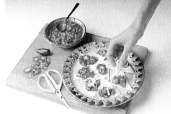

Remove from the microwave and sprinkle on ⅓ cup shredded light Monterey Jack cheese. Microwave uncovered on medium power until the cheese has melted, about 1½ minutes. (Options: Add salsa or minced peppers before sprinkling the cheese on top.)

DON'T DRESS THEM UP

When it's time to whip up your favorite breads and salads, the simpler, the better. "Try lower-fat or nonfat substitutes for those spreads and dressings," suggests Susan Kayman, Dr.P.H., consultant with the Department of Regional Health Education of the Kaiser Permanente Medical Group. She suggests using the new nonfat dressings on salads, and she recommends the fruit spreads for toast.

Thanks to advances in food science, you can enjoy delicious salad dressings that have none of the fat of those of yesteryear—or make hearty nouveau-Dagwoods that get well under 25 percent of calories from fat. And you don't have to sacrifice taste, either. Here are tactics to get flavor without the fat.

Master mayo. Everyone's a critic when it comes to mayonnaise. One person likes nonfat mayo just fine. A second accepts low-fat mayo but hates its nonfat cousin. A third simply uses low-fat or nonfat yogurt to replace mayonnaise.

If you eat chicken or tuna salad or use mayonnaise-based salad dressings, you will want to be a critic, too. Don't give up after you've tried just one taste test, says the University of California's Dr. Applegate. Try out varieties of low-fat or nonfat mayonnaise until you find one you like.

Skimp on spread. Slimming the spread on your bread is really a two-stage process—and the first step is a quantity-reduction program. In other words, use less. If you like margarine on your morning toast, let it get soft before you spread it on gauze-thin.

Jam up your bread. It's relatively easy to avoid the high-fat butter/margarine quicksand entirely. "Use jelly or marmalade or cinnamon on your toast," suggests Neal Barnard, M.D., president of the Physicians Committee for Responsible Medicine and author of *Food for Life.*

A fruit spread lets you enjoy the wake-up flavor without the fat cost, since most jams, jellies, marmalades and all-fruit spreads are virtually fat-free. (Compare that to a teaspoon of butter, which is all fat.)

Milk the fat from your milk. "It's fairly easy to go from whole milk to 2 percent milk. Going to skim milk is a little harder," says Baylor College research director Dr. Foreyt. Whole milk gets half its calories from fat, 2 percent milk is actually 35 percent fat, and skim milk is 5 percent fat. So if you sip a cup of skim instead of whole milk, you'll save 8½ fat grams a day.

Convert your cream sauce. Maybe your favorite spaghetti sauce is what some recipes call aurora—tomato sauce that's pink with a touch of cream. Substitute buttermilk (20 percent fat) or evaporated skim milk (2.3 percent fat) for the heavy cream that weighs in with 97 percent fat.

These substitutes work well in almost any cream sauce. Plus, that low-fat buttermilk lends the taste of butter to the recipe.

Give the nod to nonfat cream cheese. "It was a personal red-letter day when nonfat cream cheese came out," says Dr. Applegate. If part of your morning ritual includes having a bagel spread with cream cheese, you can eliminate the fat without missing a beat. Simply switch to the nonfat variety of cream cheese. Instead of getting ten grams of fat in a one-ounce serving (enough to cover two halves of a bagel), you'll get zero fat and just about the same flavor.

COOKING SLIM

Chefs and nutritionists have developed quite a variety of clever and easy techniques to bypass butter and oil. And every one of these tasty strategies is a major fat-slasher, since butter and oil get 100 percent of their calories from fat. To cook in style and still outwit the oil, try using some of these methods.

Sauté without the fat. Here's nutritionist Cheryl Clifford Marco's favorite

LOVE IS . . . LOW-FAT

In the What's Good for the Goose Department: A year-long study at the Fred Hutchinson Cancer Research Center in Seattle showed that husbands also benefited from their wives' low-fat menus. The research team studied 188 women on low-fat diets, counseling the women at the start on ways to introduce healthier meals to the family kitchen.

"We thought that the more trouble the women had, like making separate meals, the less successful they would be," says the cancer center's research nutritionist, Ann L. Shattuck.

But it turned out that the men ate the same low-fat meals as their wives as long as they were at home. So the husbands reaped the benefits of their wives' low-fat cooking. They wound up getting 33 percent of their calories from fat, compared to a control group of 180 men, whose diet was 37 percent fat.

technique: When a recipe calls for frying or sautéeing chopped vegetables, do it in nonfat chicken broth. Celery, onions, mushrooms and green and red peppers can all be done this way. (Any vegetable that has a high water content will cut down on the amount of oil or butter you use and also add flavor.) Use ¼ cup of chicken broth for each cup of vegetables you cook.

Even healthier for fat-free frying is vegetable broth, says Franca Alphin, R.D., nutrition director at the Duke University Diet and Fitness Center. Like chicken broth, it adds just a touch of flavor, but without any fat at all.

Add air to your oil. Every supermarket carries brand-name oil sprays. But here's a low-cost way to get your cooking spray without the propellant that is in commercial oil-spray products.

Just pour some vegetable oil into a spray bottle, suggests Cheryl Marco. Like the manufactured product, your home-made sprayer coats the pan with a micro-thin layer of oil.

"People do use less oil with a spray," adds Alphin. She offers a handy rule of thumb, too: "Remember, a second of spraying equals seven calories."

Lop off two-thirds. If you follow recipes "by the book," you may be following by the bulk as well. Often you don't need to use nearly as much oil as a fat-favoring chef recommends."I use a third as much oil as a recipe calls for. Often the taste is not affected at all," says Dr. Barnard.

Put fat on ice. You can defat store-bought chicken broth by chilling it in the refrigerator. Then, when you remove the top of the can, you'll lift off the hardened fat at the same time. You can use the same technique with homemade soups and stews. Chill in a covered container, then lift off the fat with the lid before serving.

Make nice with spice. If you have relied on the taste of butter and oils to flavor your food, and you find reduced-fat mayonnaise and plain vegetables un-

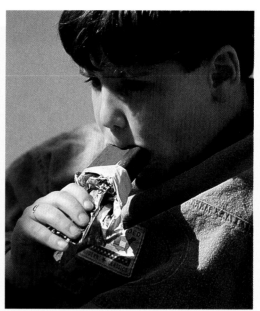

Between pack-aged snacks and other fat-packed goodies, children aged six through nine are really putting on the pudge—which may put them at risk for health problems later on.

CAUTION: CHILDREN NOSHING

The apple doesn't fall far from the tree. If Dad dines on Big Macs, Junior probably will order them, too.

But the guidelines for kids are the same as those for adults—no more than 30 percent of calories from fat for children over the age of two. Unfortunately, high-fat eating is tilting the scales toward the high end for kids, too. In a U.S. Department of Agriculture study, researchers discovered that the average diet of many elementary-school children contains 36 percent fat. (For girls, the percentages are just slightly lower.)

The National Children and Youth Fitness Study II measured 4,678 students aged six through nine and found that, in that age group, average body fat was rising. During the 20-year period that this age group was studied, researchers found that average body fat increased steadily.

"Clearly, either children are less active or they are taking in more calories. I personally think that both are happening. I think the consumption of fast foods and high-fat foods accounts for some of the rise as well," says study coauthor William Dietz, M.D., Ph.D., associate professor of pediatrics at the Tufts University School of Medicine and director of clinical nutrition at the New England Medical Center, both in Boston.

appealing at first, make like Marco Polo and look to the East. You'll find a realm of condiments, herbs and spices that can add flavor and life to your everyday menus.

Chutney, for instance. "I make a chicken salad dressing with reduced-fat mayo and nonfat yogurt and some pureed chutney," says cookbook author Ruth Spear.

The Taming of the Appetite

It's Saturday afternoon and an hour since you ate a tasty low-fat lunch—salad with your very own nonfat raspberry poppyseed dressing and a fat slice of maple bran bread, fresh from the bread machine. You're strolling Main Street, feeling fit and in control of food, exercise and life.

Then you walk by what used to be your favorite greasy spoon, and the wonderful odor of onions frying in bacon fat reaches out, grabs you by the nose and tries to pull you inside. And the odd thing is, you didn't even know you felt hungry.

What's going on?

It's appetite, and as far as your stomach is concerned, it can be a tempestuous tyrant. "You have to separate hunger from appetite. Hunger is from the stomach. Appetite is psychological," says Baylor College research director Dr. John Foreyt. In order to squelch the stomach, you have to be strong in your mind.

For starters, never let yourself get hungry. The reason is that no hunger means sharper wits. This in turn gives you the strength to squelch appetite and, with it, the evil twin that people call craving. Cravings are difficult to master, but it can be done. Here are some anti-appetite aids to get you through the worst of it.

Eat breakfast, lunch and dinner. And add a smart snack when you know you really are hungry. "Calorie-restricted diets set up a conflict between what some people call our willpower—which says eat less—and the basic biological drive (hunger) that says eat more. And this conflict has only caused a lot of eating disorders and yo-yo dieting," says Pritikin Longevity Center nutrition research specialist Dr. Jay Kenney.

Water your cells. Your appetite is wily, but it isn't smart. In fact, drown it with water and it'll think it's been fed.

DON'T CRAVE IN

You just saw a picture of the perfect pie in a food magazine, and now you can't get the thought of banana cream out of your head. You can almost taste it—flaky crust, soft sliced bananas, puffs of whipped cream. Hang on. You can ride out that food craving—quite literally—like a surfer rides out a wave.

Researchers at the University of Washington in Seattle have found that food cravings actually do cycle like waves. The craving begins, rises, peaks and eventually subsides. However, it typically takes about 20 minutes before that occurs, so it's important to be patient, advises Linda Crawford, an eating behavior specialist at Green Mountain at Fox Run, a residential weight- and health-management center for women in Ludlow, Vermont. Once the 20 minutes have passed, you're pretty much out of deep water.

To help prevent yourself from giving in to temptation and noshing when you shouldn't, it helps to engage in some activity that doesn't involve eating—like a quick walk or a bike ride—then decide how much you'll eat.

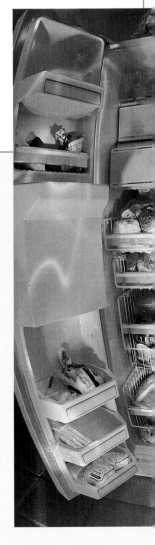

It works every time, which is why experts agree that plain water is the number-one appetite suppressant, according to diet and nutrition expert Dr. George Blackburn. Keep in mind that thirst can masquerade as hunger. That's why weight-loss experts recommend as many as eight tall glasses of water every day.

Get up and do what needs to be done. A friend just brought you some homemade Christmas cookies and your appetite is hammering away at the door of fat-resistance. You think, "I'll take them into the office so everyone else can eat them." Then you wonder, "Will those cookies survive the night?"

Yes, they will. Instead of eating the cookies before you go to bed, hem those new pants you bought. Or balance your checkbook. "Find a task you must do and do it, to get over the idea of wanting food," says Johns Hopkins weight-loss researcher Dr. Maria Simonson.

Shroud the Godiva chocolates. You bought them as a hostess gift. But you're contemplating eating a few, then probably a few more.

Instead, put the box in a brown paper bag. When Dr. Simonson's study team put all the doughnuts on a coffee cart in brown paper bags, the rate of purchase by factory workers fell by 50 percent. What works for doughnuts (about 58 percent fat) should work for chocolate (about 63 percent fat).

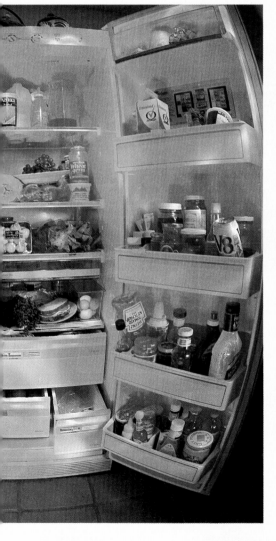

If you're a late-night eater, nip the habit at the refrigerator door with some psychological warfare. Stick some notes to the door with magnets. Weight-loss experts say the notes will be most effective if you personalize them—to stop the cravings that only you know about—but here are some ideas.

■ **CLOSED FOR THE EVENING.**

■ **BREAKFAST COMES SOON.**

■ **DRINK YOUR ICE WATER.**

■ **HAVE A MINT.**

■ **IS IT PAST YOUR SNACKTIME DEADLINE?**

■ **TOOTHPASTE YOUR PALATE.**

■ **WALK AROUND THE BLOCK THREE TIMES.**

■ **SNACKS ARE NOT SERVED HERE.**

■ **ARE YOU REALLY HUNGRY OR ARE YOU JUST BORED?**

SAY GOODNIGHT TO OVEREATING

Cravings often strike at night when a lot of people head for the bulging fridge. In fact, Dr. Simonson has catalogued three different kinds of night eaters.

■ *First, "there's the seven o'clock eater who flops down in front of the TV and munches through the evening," says Dr. Simonson.*

■ *Second is the ten o'clock eater, who says things like, "Honey, is there any of that cake left?" or "I bought some nice lemon pie." This pattern becomes a ritual, notes Dr. Simonson. The couple might even take food up to bed with them.*

■ *Third, there's the really late-night eater who "comes down to the refrigerator in the middle of the night," says Dr. Simonson. Since it takes four to six hours to digest dinner, the late-night eater may actually be hungry, she notes.*

Dr. Simonson has tips for each kind of eater.

Save dessert. *If you're a seven o'clock eater and you usually eat dessert at dinner, Dr. Simonson advises putting aside that dessert for later in the evening. Gradually cut back on the size of the portion until you can do without it, she suggests.*

Charm your mouth. *The ten o'clock eater can suck on a mint or fruit-flavored candy, says Dr. Simonson. "It helps alleviate the need for something to chew and taste," she says. If you want something to sip late at night, Dr. Simonson recommends ice water. "It can fill you up and eliminate your craving. Many people always keep a glass of ice water by the bed."*

Drink your milk. *The late-night eater who is hungry can be sated by a glass of low-fat or skim milk, according to Dr. Simonson. It's a good low-fat substitute for other late-night snacks.*

MODIFY YOUR BURGER

The main problem with hamburger is its fat content. Even if you broil three ounces of extra-lean ground beef and drain it well, you'll still get nearly 14 of your budgeted daily fat grams.

But you can balance out your fat budget if you watch your approach. Here are two neat meat strategies.

Nuke that burger. Microwaving zaps more fat from ground beef than any other cooking method, according to nutritionists—and tests have proved it. At Texas A&M University, nutritionists experimented by using various cooking methods on super-lean ground beef. They found that microwaving eliminated more of the fat in the meat than any other method.

Bulk it with beans. To bump even more fat from a helping of hamburger, replace half the meat with mashed pinto beans or black beans. You can have your usual serving but get only half the fat calories.

TRIM TACTICS

Though fat-watchers harp on the harm of hamburger, it's certainly not the only culprit. Almost any meat and poultry can be high in fat. To keep fat count to a minimum, here's how to cook by the low-fat book.

Become a better butcher. Whenever you're preparing any cut of meat, make it a habit to trim away all the visible fat. This kind of meat-tailoring is a low-fat strategy that people really stick to, according to Alan R. Kristal, Dr.P.H., who is associate researcher at the Fred Hutchinson Cancer Research Center in Seattle and also a chef. Once people get into the habit of careful carving, they don't give it up, Dr. Kristal's research has shown.

Tailor your chicken. Just follow these three easy steps to de-fat your chicken. First, take the skin off. (It's easier to remove, and makes for moister chicken, if you take off the skin after cooking.) Second, trim the visible fat under the skin. Third, don't fry it in oil.

FILL UP, NOT OUT

When you're cutting fat, you need to give vegetables, grains and pasta the same thought you give to your meat dishes. When they take center stage on your menu, they can perform like stars.

Roast 'em. For a flavorful change of pace from steamed or microwaved vegetables, try roasting them, suggests Spear. "When you oven-roast vegetables at very high heat, they caramelize and become crispy around the edges," she says.

To prepare vegetables this way, first spray a roasting pan lightly with cooking oil and set it on the bottom rack in the oven. Then place the vegetables in the pan and roast them at 450°F for 10 to 12 minutes. Vegetables that can

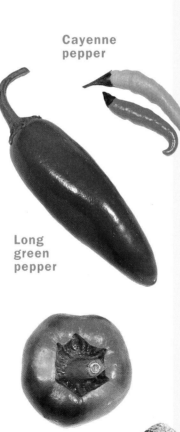

Cayenne pepper

Long green pepper

Cherry pepper

Horseradish

INCINERATE CALORIES

By choosing hot to super-hot meals, you may be able to trim some pounds.

"Whatever warms you up, slims you down," says Pritikin Longevity Center nutrition research specialist Dr. Jay Kenney. "A calorie is a unit of heat energy. When you burn calories faster, you raise your core body temperature. This helps you to eat less without feeling cold, tired or hungry."

A fiery Szechuan dinner, for example, is more calorie burning than low-spice Mandarin fare. Chili powder, chili peppers, horseradish, Tabasco and mustard all rev up our engines. So the next time you sweat when you eat, welcome the signal that your metabolism has kicked into higher gear and you're burning calories faster.

Another benefit of hot spices is their intense flavor. A spice like chili or horseradish can fill your mouth with so much taste that your appetite may be satisfied with a smaller portion, says Johns Hopkins weight-loss researcher Dr. Maria Simonson.

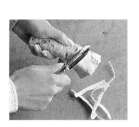

1. To prepare ground-up horseradish, re-move the leaves and clean the root with a vegetable brush to re-move the top layer of skin. Underneath is the white "meat."

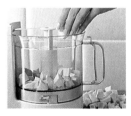

2. Chop pieces of the root and grind them in a food processor or blender. (Don't puree them.)

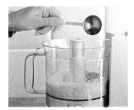

3. Add enough vinegar to moisten well.

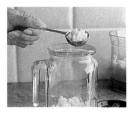

4. Place the horse-radish in a glass con-tainer with a tight-fitting lid and keep refrigerated.

be roasted include carrots and sweet potatoes (cut into large chunks), sweet red peppers, zucchini and asparagus.

Boost your main grains. There's a whole world of grains out there for the adventurous fibernaut. Many—including kasha and barley—can be found on your supermarket shelves.

Barley, which gets the Oscar for a supporting role in beef-and-barley soup, does just as well in any dish with a gen-erous sauce, such as a casserole.

Kasha is a grain widely used in the Middle East. (Here, it's sometimes called buckwheat groats.) The nutty texture complements any meal. It's a nifty, easy-to-prepare grain that you can serve like rice.

Find fiber fast. For an extra fiber bonus, have an orange (3 grams of fiber) instead of orange juice (0.2 gram of fiber), suggests Dr. Blackburn. And if

you're snacking on a bagel, make it whole wheat instead of plain, he sug-gests, because there's extra fiber in whole wheat. Another source is lentils. They not only make a hearty soup, they're also a wonderful addition to a main-dish salad.

Cook pots of pasta. Spaghetti, fettuc-cine, linguine—these are just starters in your pasta repertoire. These Italian spe-cialties can form the backbone of your high-carbohydrate, low-fat cuisine.

Reach out for some new sizes and textures. You can find pasta shaped like little ears (orrechiette), tiny radiators (radiatori) or pen points (penne). You can buy it frozen or dry—but to avoid extra fat and cholesterol, don't eat pasta that's made with eggs.

Pasta also comes in a variety of tanta-lizing flavors, each suggested by a dif-ferent color.

DOES HASTE MAKE WAIST?

You're sopping up tomato sauce with the last heel of bread. Then it's gone and your plate is clean; there's nothing left. You glance around the table. Your dinner companions are all still eating—lingering over their linguine.

A voice may be telling you, "Slow down, you eat too fast." But what difference does it really make if you clean your plate too quickly?

In a study at the Univer-sity of Pennsylvania in Philadelphia, researchers had 18 women—9 lean and 9 obese—eat sandwiches and bagels that were cut up into different sizes. The re-searchers found that there was a wide range of eating speeds among both groups—and no evidence that obese people eat any faster than those at normal weight.

This contradicts what di-etitians and doctors have be-lieved since 1962, when re-search first showed that lean people eat less because they eat more slowly than obese people.

But there's no doubt that people who take time to re-ally taste and enjoy their food are less likely to gulp it down.

"It takes the brain 20 min-utes to get the message from the stomach," says Susan Olson, Ph.D., director of psychological services and clinical psychologist at the Southwest Bariatric Nutri-tion Center in Scottsdale, Arizona. In other words, you may get full before you know it, unless you're taking the time to relish your meal. So sit back, eat slowly and enjoy your food, Dr. Olson suggests.

Move Over, Drastic Diets

Okay, eat as much as you want, until you're full.

Good eating topped the list when 6,000 *Prevention* readers described how they lost weight and kept it off. Many had personalized plans that deftly combined low-fat eating with regular exercise. They described how they created new, great-tasting favorite meals and snacks by using low-fat ingredients. They sang the praises of low-fat mayo, skinless chicken, lean turkey breast and no-oil cooking.

Best of all were the foods they described—grainy, delicious oatmeal bread, chewy brown-rice salad, delicious pasta, pineapple chunks with nonfat vanilla yogurt, roasted vegetables and much more.

For many of us, the concept of "eat as much as you want" seems to defy all the traditional laws of dieting. When so many authorities have been saying for so many years that you have to starve to lose weight, it's hard to believe otherwise.

But remember, the studies in weight loss are now tilted in favor of eating—the right way.

"All our studies show that you can eat as much as you want if it's low-fat," says Cornell University researcher and professor Dr. David Levitsky.

Anyone who's been reading about diets—or trying one after another—might find it hard to believe that weight loss could be so straightforward. But research keeps pointing to that conclusion.

In one of Dr. Levitsky's studies, for instance, he followed 13 women as they alternated between low-fat and regular diets. Except for the fat content, the food in both diets was the same. The women ate normal foods that required no-fuss preparation, like pasta with vegetables, chicken-rice casserole and pizza. They choose their own portion sizes,

too. But in one phase of the study they ate foods that were prepared using low-fat ingredients or nonfat cooking methods. In another phase, they had the same foods prepared with traditional high-fat ingredients like whole milk, butter, cream and the usual cooking oils.

Here's what happened. When they ate low-fat, the 13 women steadily lost ½ pound a week. And they said that substituting low-fat for high-fat ingredients and methods didn't make a smidgen of difference. The weight loss was so painless, the women weren't even aware they were "dieting."

"We encourage people to eat till they feel full," says Dr. Levitsky. You really don't have to restrain yourself, he points out, because your body will do it for you.

But how?

Dr. Levitsky explains: Our body's "receptors," the nerve endings that tell us whether or not we're full, are attuned to carbohydrates, not fat. In other words, if we eat a large helping of spaghetti or a big slice of bread, which both have lots of carbohydrates, our body's receptors say, "You're full!" But they don't signal anything at all if we overdo on a salad drowned in oily dressing that's nearly all fat. So you need the carbohydrates, but not the fat, in order to feel like you've had plenty to eat.

"As you lower the fat, more and more carbohydrates come in, and your body will regulate them," Dr. Levitsky explains. Even when you're eating as much as you want, you'll be getting fewer calories. And since you can increase the volume of food, you won't feel deprived and crave food. As a result, you'll lose weight without ever being hungry.

HOW THEY DID IT

When 6,000 *Prevention* readers told us how they lost weight—and how they keep it off—they repeated many of the tips that we have heard from weight-loss experts. Not surprisingly, low-fat eating and exercise topped the tip sheet.

Here's what folks do:

■ 97 percent of the readers exercise.

■ 96 percent stick to low-fat eating.

■ 92 percent read food labels when they choose their food.

■ 91 percent eat no sweets.

■ 89 percent cut calories in general.

■ 83 percent eat high-fiber foods.

■ 79 percent choose vegetables and light meals over red meat.

■ 79 percent use meal planning.

■ 58 percent defat their recipes.

Other popular strategies include drinking more water, keeping problem foods out of the house and keeping a food diary.

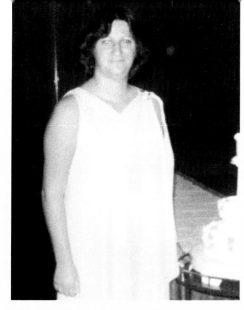

THE FAYE WAY
TO WEIGHT LOSS

At the age of 33, Karen Faye weighed 220 pounds and her cholesterol was over 300. Working third shift as a nurse in an intensive care unit, she frequently saw heart attack victims. And many of them were overweight. "I saw the writing on the artery walls," she says. "I said to myself, 'I'm going to die before I'm 50.'"

Karen knew that cutting fat from her diet—in addition to a daily exercise program—was the key.

Her goal was to lose 80 pounds, but Karen says, "I took it one day and one step at a time." Within six months she had lost 50 pounds. By sticking to a low-fat diet and continuing to exercise, she eventually reached her goal.

Ten years after starting her weight-loss program, and 80 pounds lighter, Karen Faye won the title of "Mrs. Physical Fitness" in the Mrs. United States championship.

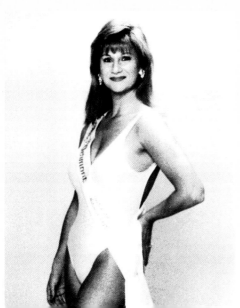

SEVEN DAYS THAT PAY

If you're wondering how to get started on a weight-loss plan, here's what experts recommend as a starter set—a whole week's worth of sample food swaps and weight-loss activities. Hold to this for just a week, and you'll naturally trim fat without a backward glance.

SUNDAY
- Eat roast turkey breast instead of pot roast.
- Have angel food cake instead of cheesecake.
- Drink fizzy, fruit-flavored water instead of soda.

MONDAY
- Have a new breakfast—a fat-free bran muffin and a glass of 1 percent milk instead of a Danish and whole milk.
- Use the stairs at work instead of the elevator.

TUESDAY
- Use nonfat Italian dressing on your lunchtime salad.
- Have cracked-wheat bread instead of french fries.
- Have an apple for a snack instead of a candy bar.
- Go out for a two-mile stroll.

WEDNESDAY
- Have one slice of cheese pizza and nonfat frozen yogurt for lunch instead of two slices of pepperoni pizza.
- Have vegetarian fat-free chili and fat-free whole-wheat crackers for dinner instead of beef chili and tortilla chips.

THURSDAY
- Use nonfat cream cheese on your breakfast bagel instead of regular cream cheese.
- Snack on light microwave popcorn instead of potato chips.

FRIDAY
- Sweat it out during lunch in a low-impact aerobics class.
- Have a couple of club sodas instead of a couple of beers at happy hour.

SATURDAY
- Go for a bike ride.
- Picnic on tuna sandwiches made with nonfat mayonnaise and serve three-bean salad instead of potato salad.
- For dessert, have gingersnaps Instead of chocolate chip cookies.

NOTES
- Take along an apple in case you get hungry.
- Keep a water bottle handy.

Gut-Level Relief for Digestive Woes

E at, drink and be merry. For some people, it's a way of life. But there are times when festive feasting can make the merriest souls misanthropic. The sight of salsa, the crunch of crackers or the mention of milk summons waves of dread. That's the way people react when they have a digestive disorder—when what goes down might come up . . . or worse.

Tummy troubles read like a who's who of gastrointestinal bad guys. There's common constipation, ubiquitous ulcers, galling gallstones and unflattering flatulence. Other problems include celiac disease (the inability to digest an ingredient found in grains), inflammatory bowel disease (which attacks the lining and walls of the intestine) and diverticulitis (infection of pouches in the colon wall that can occur over time).

And if the enigma of your innards confuses you, don't worry. You're not alone.

"The digestive system is a very big subject that confuses patients all the time—it confuses doctors, too," confides William B. Ruderman, M.D., chairman of the Department of Gastroenterology at the Cleveland Clinic Florida and a staff doctor for the Cleveland Clinic Hospital and Broward General Hospital, all in Fort Lauderdale.

According to the National Institutes of Health (NIH) in Bethesda, Mary-land, more than 20 million Americans—1 out of every 13 of us—have a chronic digestive disease. Each day digestive woes cause more than 19 million absences from work. Each year they claim 191,000 lives (including deaths from stomach cancer), cost $40 billion in direct medical costs and cause 35 million doctor visits.

THE UNMUNCHABLES

Your digestive tract normally works inconspicuously, like a stagehand working the curtain at a play. It's this low profile that causes some people to forget about digestion. They'll eat everything from Jorge's Hot Jalapeño Dip to Mom's apple pie and let nature take its course.

But if you have a digestive disorder, it's not this easy. Food can become an enemy, not an ally. Many gastrointestinal diseases require medical treatment. Since so many conditions are complex and symptoms can't be self-diagnosed, you'll probably need a doctor's exam before you can begin to get a grip on what's ailing you. Moreover, you should certainly consult a doctor before making any radical changes in your diet. Then you can take some important food-focused steps to help ease or reverse your problems. After all, it's you who chooses your daily menu—and by pointing your fork in the right direction, you also point the way toward feeling better.

DIGESTION FROM START TO FINISH

The digestive system is a tube about 30 feet long, with numerous twists, turns and detours. It's made up of about a dozen parts, each one playing an integral role in digestion. The stars of the show are the stomach and intestines, but a strong supporting cast includes the tongue, esophagus, gallbladder, liver and pancreas.

Digestion begins with the first bite, as saliva breaks down food. After swallowing, wavelike muscle contractions force the food to the stomach. Then contractions in the stomach move the food into the small intestine, where nutrients are absorbed. Finally, the food is moved to the large intestine, where salts and water are absorbed, and from there leftover waste goes into the rectum.

On average, the digestive tract handles 1 quart of saliva, about 2 quarts of food and drink, 1 quart of bile, 2 quarts of stomach juices and 1½ quarts of pancreatic juices every day.

Esophagus. *This collapsible, muscular tube, which is about ten inches long, lies behind your windpipe. It moves food to your stomach in one to eight seconds.*

Stomach. *This J-shaped sac at the end of your esophagus is about the size of a large sausage when empty. It stores and digests food, then empties it into the small intestine in two to six hours.*

Liver. *Weighing about four pounds, it lies under the diaphragm in the upper right side of your chest. The liver produces bile to help digest fats.*

Pancreas. *Lying behind the J-curve of your stomach, the six-inch pancreas is attached to your small intestine. It secretes enzymes that digest food and regulate blood sugar.*

Small intestine. *Averaging 21 feet in length, this part of the digestive tract does the lion's share of digestion. Inside, it's covered with four to five million microscopic projections called villi that absorb food.*

Large intestine. *This 5-foot length of the intestinal tract passes indigestible waste from the small intestine to the rectum. Some liquid and minerals are reabsorbed through the intestinal walls.*

Gallbladder. *A small, pear-shaped sac along the underside of your liver, your gallbladder stores bile, which it gets from the liver. Bile is squeezed into the small intestine during meals.*

If you have a digestive disorder, whether it's diarrhea or diverticular disease, you don't have to say farewell to delightful dining. But you do need to deal with the problem, and that may take a slight adjustment of attitude.

View your body as a machine and food as its fuel, suggests Betty Garrity, R.D., an outpatient dietitian at the University of California Medical Center at San Diego. "Your body has to receive the correct fuel to function properly," Garrity says. Just as your car might sputter when you fill it with low-grade gasoline, your body—and digestive tract—might react to low-grade food, she says.

Although gastric flare-ups occur for many reasons—and not all are diet related—Garrity notes you can make these maladies more tolerable (or wipe them out completely) by watching what you eat.

Dr. Ruderman emphasizes that you don't need to monitor every single item that's on your menu—just be aware of what you eat. "I don't think you have to be a food faddist or a nut case to watch your diet," he says. "It just makes prudent common sense."

Here's how dietary direction and midsection monitoring can help you soothe your gurgling gut.

HEARTBURN: WHEN THE INSIDES ACT UP

It's one thing to have a heart that yearns, but it's another to have a heart that burns.

Heartburn doesn't threaten the heart, but it can certainly be painful. Most people experience it as a sudden burning sensation in the chest that often occurs soon after a meal.

"Everybody has heartburn once in a while. It's that widespread," says Samuel Meyers, M.D., clinical professor of medicine at Mount Sinai School of Medicine in New York.

But even though it's as common as checked pants on a golf course, that burning sensation in the chest can be scary. "It's not unusual for people to wind up in the emergency room because they think it's a heart attack, when in truth they just have heartburn," Dr. Meyers says.

Given the fact that as many as 25 million Americans get heartburn daily, it's lucky this everyday problem comes from a turbulent tummy rather than a tired ticker. It's also good that, for most who get it, the discomfort usually ends within two hours.

Heartburn occurs in the lower esophagus when digestive juices wash back from the stomach—a process called reflux. The mixture carries stomach acid and bile, which can burn the delicate mucous lining of your esophagus. Normally, a sphincter muscle between the esophagus and the stomach acts like a one-way valve, letting food in and preventing reflux. When this muscle weakens or relaxes, heartburn occurs. Since you can't pinpoint the location of the burning sensation, heartburn feels like it's just somewhere in your chest.

Treating heartburn at home can be easy. For starters, doctors recommend that you stand up or take a stroll after eating to let gravity go to work. (If you lie down after a meal, you're just asking for trouble.) And for smokers, the first step toward quelling heartburn is to give up the nicotine habit, since nicotine helps stimulate acid production and impairs the sphincter muscle that controls reflux.

Apart from those tactics, doctors suggest that you take a good look at what you put on your plate. Many heartburn sufferers think spicy foods are the only ones to avoid. But according to doctors, it's not just people who binge on Mexican buffets who suffer. Here are other food factors to consider if you want to prevent a reflux revolt.

Spurn the burn. Chocolate, peppermint, coffee, alcohol and fried or fatty foods can relax the sphincter muscle at the end of your esophagus.

Among the high-fat foods that may fire up heartburn are roasted almonds (24 grams of fat per ¼ cup) avocados (9 grams per ¼ avocado), spareribs (26 grams per three-ounce serving), premium ice cream (12 grams per ½ cup) and fried, breaded onion rings (16 grams per three ounces or eight or nine rings).

An after-dinner mint or chocolate, a cup of coffee or a nightcap may be exactly what you don't need. Doctors say these typical postmeal treats—almost a ritual for some people—are known firestarters for anyone prone to heartburn.

Take away acid additions. Highly acidic foods add to heartburn by increasing the acidity in your stomach. Hot and cold beverages—including coffee, tea and some juices—are among the acid culprits.

"Apple, orange, grape and tomato juice are all very concentrated and can

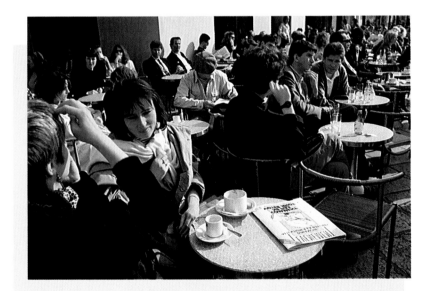

COFFEE, TEA OR HEARTBURN?

Here's a hot tip about drinking coffee—or any other hot beverage: Let it cool. Researchers at England's Manchester Royal Infirmary found that people who drank very hot beverages had higher risk of heartburn than those who let their drinks cool. According to these findings, people who preferred their tea and coffee in the temperature range of 143°F were more likely to have the problem than those who had hot drinks in the 132° range. (Average bathwater, by comparison, is 114°.) Researchers suspect the hot liquid breaks down the protective mucous lining of the digestive system, making it susceptible to heartburn.

injure the esophagus if you already have heartburn," says Dr. Meyers.

Take a water break. Sipping water after a meal dilutes acid in your esophagus, according to Dr. Meyers. Several glasses after each meal should bring quick relief.

"The esophagus is not made to handle reflux. If you don't water it down, it'll burn the esophagus, like acid burns your skin," he explains.

IBS: TAMING YOUR CRANKY COLON

Irritable bowel syndrome is one gastrointestinal disease that travels under many aliases. Called IBS for short, it's also known as colitis, spastic colon and spastic bowel. The usual symptoms of IBS include cramps, diarrhea and constipation.

IBS is common. In one study of 803 70-year-old Danish men and women, doctors found that 18 percent of the men and 32 percent of the women had at least two of the three marker symptoms of irritable bowel.

Despite its commonness, IBS is confounding because doctors don't know what causes or cures it. They do suspect, however, that nerves, stress and diet may bring on the symptoms.

A case in point: In one British study researchers asked 36 people with IBS to picture a peacefully flowing river that represented their digestive system working the way it should. After four 40-minute sessions of self-hypnosis over seven weeks, 20 of the patients reported improvements. Eleven of them, ended up with no symptoms at all.

But a problem that's so widespread and that springs from unknown causes is sometimes difficult to diagnose, Dr. Meyers says.

"What it usually boils down to is simply asking the patient the right questions and then listening sympathetically," he notes.

When you have IBS, your large intestine contracts spasmodically at the slightest provocation. Sometimes medi-

cines and foods are at fault, while at other times it's stress and emotions.

Fortunately, you can fight IBS fairly well with dietary and lifestyle changes.

Watch milk and its ilk. Milk and dairy products contain a hard-to-digest sugar, called lactose, that can aggravate an irritable bowel in some people. "There is a high incidence of lactose intolerance in people with irritable bowel syndrome," cautions Marvin Schuster, M.D., professor of medicine and psychiatry at Johns Hopkins Bayview Medical Center and chief of digestive diseases at Francis Scott Key Medical Center, both in Baltimore. He estimates that up to 40 percent of people with irritable bowel syndrome have difficulty with dairy products.

Cut the fat and protein. Most high-fat foods contain a lot of protein as well as fat—and that's significant because both stimulate gastrointestinal secretions and muscle contractions. While these reactions are normal, they may aggravate IBS, doctors say.

High-fat foods include dairy products like whole milk and butter, fatty meats and any products that contain oil. You can quickly find out how much fat is in packaged, canned or frozen foods by reading the new food labels. And any time you choose fresh vegetables, lean meat or fish and skim milk products, you're on a fat-slashing path. But remember, even lean meats and skim milk contain protein that can stimulate secretions.

Serve smaller portions. Every time you eat, nerve impulses make your large intestine contract. The more you eat, the more they contract as your body prepares for digestion.

With IBS, more contractions may mean more symptoms. Since you can't possibly stop eating to avoid this reaction, doctors recommend that you eat your food in smaller portions so your insides are less stimulated.

You can do this by eating less food more often. For example, instead of *(continued on page 72)*

The Ins and Outs of Fiber

Imagine you're living in prehistoric times and you're hungry. For dinner, you can pick fruits and vegetables, or you can hunt a tenacious hairy mastodon. What do you do?

That's sort of how early humans got so much fiber. It's estimated that early hunter-gatherers got 65 percent of their food from plants, probably because the plants didn't fight back.

While life is different now, our fiber consumption has suffered at the hands of progress. Today we can roll through a drive-through and get a hot meal in less time than it takes to say *Paleozoic*. But while you may get your meal faster, you'll get less fiber.

And that's too bad, because fiber can go a long way in placating many digestive disorders.

Fortunately, you don't have to become a hunter-gatherer throwback to make sure you get adequate fiber. Just take advantage of fresh produce in the nearest supermarket, where you'll find enough fiber to prevent constipation, diarrhea, irritable and inflamed bowels and other gastrointestinal problems such as diverticulosis and diverticulitis. Fiber helps discourage other problems as well—from irritations like hemorrhoids to major-league diseases like colon cancer.

"When it comes to fiber, Americans

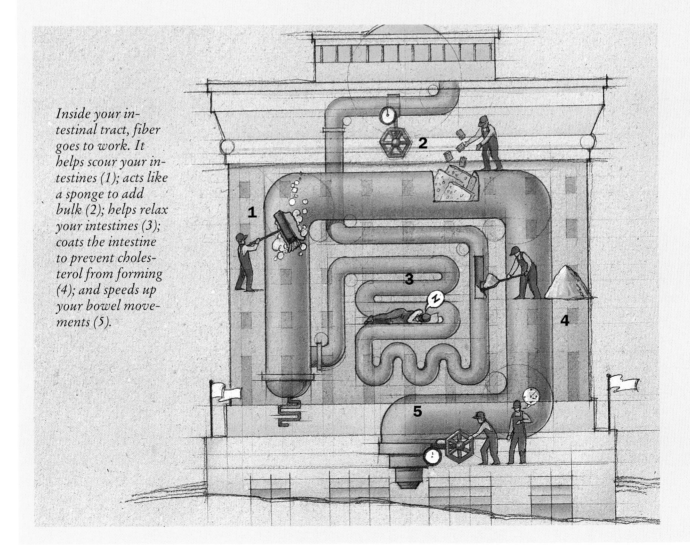

Inside your intestinal tract, fiber goes to work. It helps scour your intestines (1); acts like a sponge to add bulk (2); helps relax your intestines (3); coats the intestine to prevent cholesterol from forming (4); and speeds up your bowel movements (5).

TARGET YOUR HEALTH

You can easily get the 20 to 35 grams of fiber that doctors say you need for super digestion by making sure your daily diet includes about five servings of fruits or vegetables and six servings of whole-grain breads, cereals or legumes. (Consider an apple or ½ cup of whole-grain cereal as one serving.)

Here are first-rate fiber sources to help you make your goal.

0–3.5 g.
Brussels sprouts (½ cup)
Sweet potato (1)
Orange (1)
Apple (1)

3.6–4.3 g.
Pear (1)
Raisins (½ cup)
Oatmeal (¾ cup)
Wheat germ (¼ cup toasted)

4.4–6 g.
Raspberries (1 cup)
Whole-wheat spaghetti (1 cup)
Artichoke (½ cup boiled)
Barley (½ cup)

6.1–7 g.
Chick-peas (½ cup)
Kidney beans (½ cup)
Lima beans (½ cup)
Oat bran (½ cup)
Black beans (½ cup)

on the whole are probably worse off than many other countries because we're so industrialized," says University of California dietitian Betty Garrity. She points out that our industrialized society gives us more opportunities to avoid fiber by indulging in fast food and processed foods.

You need both types of fiber—soluble and insoluble—doctors say, to help keep your digestive tract on track. Soluble fiber dissolves in water and forms a gel that coats your insides. It's found in fruits and also in beans and grains. Oats, barley and rye are among the best sources of soluble fiber.

Insoluble fiber acts like a sponge, soaking up water and making stool softer, heavier and more easily passed. It also speeds up digestion. There are many good vegetable sources, as well as cereals and wheat, as you can see from the fiber target on this page.

If you're like most people, you probably get 10 to 15 grams of fiber a day, or about as much as you'd get by eating three to five apples. That's a far cry from the 20 to 35 grams most doctors and researchers agree are optimal for digestive health.

Yet with all the cheerleading for fiber, it's amazing that just a few decades ago, many experts considered it virtually useless. Doctors knew it added bulk, but they couldn't figure out how it provided any nutritional benefit. Now our attitude toward fiber has done an about-face.

"Fiber definitely is big in the study of digestive disorders," says Dr. Marvin Schuster of Johns Hopkins Bayview Medical Center and Francis Scott Key Medical Center. Fiber is important, he says, precisely because it bulks up the stool. And this bulking action, by taking pressure off the inside of the intestine, helps prevent problems like diverticulosis.

Even though you might not get a full 35 grams of fiber a day, remember that anything you do to increase your fiber is a step in the right direction, adds Dr. Schuster. Here's a starter set of bulk-building tactics.

Give chick-peas a chance. Chick-peas (also called garbanzo beans or ceci) are one of the best sources of fiber around. Each half cup carries seven grams of fiber, about as much as you'd get in two big apples. Use chick-peas generously as an addition to rice dishes, salad or even chili.

Even though they're convenient, avoid canned chick-peas, because salt often gets added during processing. To prepare dry chick-peas, wash them thoroughly. Then cover with water

(continued)

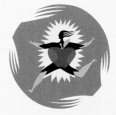

and soak overnight. Drain, add new water and cook for about 2½ hours, until soft. (You can freeze the leftovers; they'll keep for about four months.)

Don't shed your spud's skin. Next time you have KP duty, leave the skin on the potatoes—then eat them skin and all. "The skin of the potato is an excellent source of fiber," Garrity says.

Compare the four grams of total dietary fiber provided by an average baked potato (with skin) to the nearly two grams of fiber in the same size raw potato.

Keep the fiber wrapping on your

fruit. "Keep the skins on fruits, too. They're all more beneficial that way," Garrity says.

The skin of one apple alone contributes about half a gram—or about 20 percent—of its total dietary fiber.

Compare apples and oranges. And they can be compared—as long as you're talking about fiber. Both have about three grams of dietary fiber. And pears are even higher: They have over four grams.

Beef up on oat bran. A great way to boost fiber is to eat more bran. Its soluble fiber forms a kind of gel as it passes through your digestive system,

MAKE THE SWITCH TO FIBER

You can turn an old fiber-poor diet into a new fiber-rich one. And if you do, there's little threat of dietary boredom, since many healthful and tasty foods are high in fiber. The table below shows how you can get 27 grams more fiber in your diet with just a few food swaps. (The fiber amounts listed are for standard serving sizes.)

Old Menu		New Menu	
FOOD	**FIBER (G.)**	**FIBER (G.)**	**FOOD**
Breakfast			
Orange juice	*0.1*	*3.1*	*Orange*
Corn flakes	*0.5*	*9.0*	*High-fiber cereal*
Doughnut	*trace*	*2.1*	*Whole-wheat toast*
Lunch			
Hamburger (on white bun)	*0.7*	*4.6*	*Chili*
French fries	*3.1*	*3.4*	*Sweet potato, baked*
Dinner			
Lettuce salad	*1.4*	*6.1*	*Lettuce salad with chick-peas, broccoli and mushrooms*
Chicken	*trace*	*trace*	*Chicken*
White rice	*0.2*	*1.7*	*Brown rice*
Snacks			
Apple	*3.0*	*4.3*	*Pear*
Potato chips	*1.0*	*2.7*	*Popcorn*
TOTAL	**10.0**	**37.0**	

BREAKTHROUGHS IN HEALING

1 8 2 0 – 3 0

Sylvester Graham travels the East Coast extolling his fiber cookie, the Graham cracker. Defying the doctors of the time, Graham believed that fiber was good for you.

1 9 6 6

Surgeon Captain Cleave of Britain publishes *The Saccharine Disease*, which claims that many of the diseases in Western culture are related to the consumption of refined carbohydrates. This sparks the modern interest in fiber and serves as the basis for studies in the 1970s.

1 9 7 2 – 7 6

British researchers Hugh C. Trowell and Denis P. Burkitt link high-fiber diets in Africans to low cholesterol and low incidence of colon cancer. Experts begin to realize that fiber, which remains largely undigested, is critically important to digestive health.

1 9 8 5

For the first time, the U.S. Department of Agriculture surveys Americans to find out how much fiber they get in their daily diet. Results show that adults get only one-third to one-half of the 35 grams recommended by most doctors.

slowing the rate of food absorption.

Oat bran comes in raw, powdered form—which gives you a concentrated two grams of dietary fiber in two tablespoons. But there are tastier ways to get this type of bran. Oatmeal, for instance, provides nearly four grams per ¾-cup serving, and if you add fruits and nuts to your morning bowl of oatmeal, you'll get even more.

Pick a peck of pectin. Another good source of gel-forming soluble fiber is pectin, which is found in many fruits, including apples, apricots and grapefruit, and some vegetables. Since pectin gels so easily in water, you help smooth out the digestive process every time you eat a high-pectin fruit salad, snack on dried apricots or eat a grapefruit for breakfast.

Wheat is neat, too. On the other side of bran land—wheat instead of oats—is insoluble fiber, which absorbs water and increases in bulk. Insoluble fiber is jam-packed into wheat bran, and it's also found in vegetables. Because it "bulks up" by absorbing water inside the digestive tract, it's particularly good for preventing constipation.

Wheat bran has a generous three grams of dietary fiber for every two tablespoons—as much as in a whole apple.

One caution, however: In a study of 100 outpatients at the University Hospital of South Manchester in Manchester, England, doctors found that 55 percent of those with IBS got worse when they had lots of whole-meal wheat and bran products in their diet,

while only 10 percent improved.

You can get a good dose of wheat bran from many breakfast cereals. One bowl (⅓ cup) of Nabisco 100% Bran, for example, has 9 grams of fiber, while ½ cup of General Mills Fiber One has 14 grams.

Do the (micro) wave. The microwave oven can be a powerful ally in your quest for more fiber. Microwave cooking takes just minutes, so fruits and vegetables keep their fibrous makeup better than they do in conventional cooking. "The microwave really preserves fiber in the foods better," Garrity says.

To microwave vegetables, set your microwave oven on High and cook quickly. The vegetables should still be firm, but cooked.

HIGH-FIBER, NO-FIRE CHILI

Here's a quick and simple recipe for a mild chili that's guaranteed to boost your fiber by ten grams per serving—that's as much as ½ cup of bran or three apples.

If you want meat, add eight ounces of extra-lean ground beef. (Crumble it into the saucepan before sautéing the vegetables and brown it over medium heat. Add peppers, onions and oil, then continue with the recipe.)

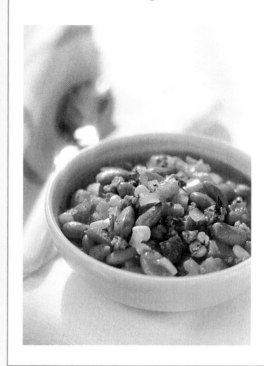

2	cups diced sweet red or green peppers
1½	cups diced onions
1	tablespoon olive oil
1	clove garlic, minced
1	tablespoon chili powder
1	teaspoon ground cumin
½	teaspoon dried oregano
1	can (28 ounces) whole tomatoes, with juice
½	cup defatted chicken stock
½	cup mild salsa
1	can (19 ounces) kidney beans, rinsed and drained
1½	cups frozen corn

In a 3-quart saucepan over medium heat, sauté the peppers and onions in the oil for 5 minutes, or until softened. Stir in the garlic, chili powder, cumin and oregano. Stir for 1 minute.

Add the tomatoes and juice. With a large spoon, break up the tomatoes. Stir in the stock and salsa and bring to a boil. Simmer for 10 minutes, stirring to prevent sticking.

Add the beans and corn. Cook, stirring often, for 10 minutes, or until thickened.

Makes 4 servings.

Per serving: 290 calories, 5.6 g. fat (17% of calories), 10 g. dietary fiber, 0 mg. cholesterol, 442 mg. sodium.

three squares a day, try eating six half-meals to keep your colon calm.

IBD: WHEN FOOD FEEDS PAIN

Inflammatory bowel disease (IBD) is a generic term for a group of digestive disorders that may affect as many as two million people, but generally it applies to ulcerative colitis and Crohn's disease.

Ulcerative colitis is what happens when the lining of your large intestine becomes inflamed. It's more likely to be a problem for younger people: Of the quarter-million Americans who have ulcerative colitis, nearly all are between the ages of 15 and 40.

Crohn's disease is an inflammation involving all layers of the intestinal walls. Though it usually affects the small and large intestine, Crohn's can disturb the large one alone. Doctors suspect Crohn's may be linked to problems in the immune system.

The symptoms associated with Crohn's include abdominal pain, weight loss and diarrhea. With ulcerative colitis, some symptoms are similar, but you can also expect bloody diarrhea.

Some people have symptom-free periods, but even then, doctors warn, IBD should always be treated, because it can lead to rectal bleeding, fever and even death. And in children, untreated IBD can cause stunted growth.

Doctors don't know what causes IBD or how to cure it, and there's not much you can do diet-wise to help.

"I usually tell people to eat whatever they like. However, during acute attacks, while low-fiber and low-lactose diets may not reduce inflammation, they may make you more comfortable," says Dr. Meyers.

Dr. Ruderman of the Cleveland Clinic also warns against getting too much fiber during severe bouts of IBD. "With a high-fiber diet and IBD, you could have more cramps, especially when the bowel is harmed by disease," he says.

For those who have IBD, the toughest part is just adjusting to living with it. You need to stay in touch with your doctor—and it might be helpful to talk to others who have the same problem. Ask your doctor for information about the Crohn's and Colitis Foundation of America, which helps keep people informed about IBD.

NAUSEA: STOPPING THAT GREEN FEELING

When that endearing *Sesame Street* personality Kermit the Frog sang "It's Not Easy Being Green," he was reciting more than just an aphorism for amphibians. He could have been pining about nausea.

DON'T BLAME THE BOSS FOR ULCERS

In our society, ulcers once were seen as perverse badges of honor. If you were overworked, people said, you got an ulcer—period. But now research has shown that the work/ulcer connection is much overrated. Instead, the leading villains are bacteria and some medications such as aspirin.

Ulcers are like little wounds on the inside of your stomach or the upper part of your lower intestine. Two types are most common. Duodenal (pronounced *doo-oh-DEE-nel*) ulcers form when gastric juices—originating in the stomach—burn parts of your duodenum, the first part of your small intestine. Stomach ulcers affect almost a million of us each year. They form when the stomach's resistance to digestive juices breaks down.

In some cases, bacteria play a part in causing ulcers. *Helicobacter pylori* (*H. pylori*, for short) is a type of microscopic S-shaped bacteria that can live undetected in your stomach's mucous lining for years. These bacteria are associated with ulcers in about 15 percent of the people who are infected.

Doctors have known about the association between *H. pylori* and ulcers for a number of years, but they still do not have enough evidence to say that the bacteria cause ulcers. They have shown, however, that eradicating the bacteria with antibiotics heals the ulcer.

These findings also change long-held beliefs about the need for a bland diet for those with ulcers. Doctors have found that diet therapy—which used to be prescribed for ulcers—just doesn't work as a cure. Some foods, however, may help.

Nausea is queasiness that usually comes before vomiting. The word is derived from a Greek word meaning "seasickness," which is a type of nausea caused by the disruption of your body's balance control center.

But we all know that nausea doesn't just happen on the high seas. "Nausea is very nonspecific—you can get it from a lot of things," Dr. Ruderman says. As he points out, you may feel nauseated when your body reacts to something you've been drinking (alcohol, for instance) or when bacteria irritate your insides—one signal of food poisoning. Even raging hormones can cause nausea, as happens when pregnant women have morning sickness.

But whatever the cause, here's how you can eat to ease your stomach.

Put the bite on nausea. Eating a little bit of food during nausea may sound as if you're throwing fuel on the fire, but it can actually help calm your stomach's contractions.

"Sometimes it helps to eat something bland, like plain crackers or dry toast," Dr. Ruderman says.

But if you do nibble on these mild munchies, skip the butter or margarine. Any kind of fatty spread is harder to digest and can make things worse.

Or take five. Hours, that is, and do nothing. "Sometimes it's best to keep the stomach empty and not eat or drink anything for four to six hours," Dr. Ruderman says. But at the end of that rest time, you should start feeling better. And if nausea leads to vomiting, Dr. Ruderman warns, you may need to take some other steps—especially if the vomiting continues for a while.

"If you go 12 to 24 hours without being able to keep anything down, you're going to get into trouble. Dehydration is just around the corner," he adds. When nausea and vomiting persist and fluids won't stay down for this long, you should check with your doctor, Dr. Ruderman advises.

Go gingerly. Studies show that an old-fashioned nausea remedy, ginger, can sometimes work even better than over-the-counter drugs.

"My mother always told me to drink ginger ale because ginger has a beneficial effect on nausea," says Philip Miner, M.D., professor of medicine at the University of Kansas Medical Center in Kansas City.

While ginger ale has only a small dose of ginger, you get a mightier punch from ginger in capsule form. If you know you're likely to get carsick, airsick or seasick, some doctors suggest that you try taking two or three 550-milligram ginger capsules 15 minutes before traveling. On a long trip, take another dose after four hours or so.

Or start your journey—by land, sea or air—with a cup of soothing ginger tea, which can be just as effective for some people. Powdered ginger capsules and ginger teas are widely available at health food stores.

FOOD POISONING: BANNING THE BACTERIA

A summertime picnic is a romantic notion, but if you get careless with the egg salad, it will set your stomach in motion.

When we're getting ready for picnics, barbecues or big family dinners, we sometimes handle food in ways that allow it to become contaminated. And that can lead to food poisoning, which affects more than 24 million of us each year.

Food poisoning occurs when you swallow bacteria. Once inside, they either burrow into the walls of your intestine or dump bacteria-size waste that harms your gut.

Normally our bodies destroy bacteria during digestion, but when we can't kill the germs, we sometimes get sick. Symptoms typically include nausea, vomiting and diarrhea, all of which usually go away in a few days.

But many episodes of food poisoning can be avoided. It's just a matter of using common sense when you're handling and preparing your delectable delights, says dietitian Betty Garrity of the University of California.

Here's how to ward off the bacteria that would like to bug your insides.

Avoid the raw deals. Whether you're dining out, picnicking or shopping for dinner, watch out for the raw foods that are notorious villains. These include shellfish such as oysters, mussels and clams, sushi and steak tartare. "These types of raw foods definitely can increase your risk of food poisoning," Dr. Ruderman says.

Also, you should be aware that some restaurants still make Caesar salad with raw eggs, even though there's a risk of getting stomach-churning salmonella bacteria from uncooked eggs. If you're dining out, leave Caesar to history—unless you find out how the chef prepares the salad.

Don't lose your temperature. It's important to keep foods at the right temperature, or else they can become a nasty breeding ground for germs.

"This is mostly common sense. Keep hot foods hot, cold foods cold," says Dr. Meyers of Mount Sinai School of Medicine. Watch out for foods that are poorly handled, incompletely cooked or precooked and then warmed, he stresses. He suggests warming up foods to at least 140°F—which you can check with a food thermometer. And make sure the food is heated through, not just on the outside. Any stored food should be kept below 40°. Basically that just means keeping food in the refrigerator, where the temperature is usually 34° to 40°.

Watch the doggy bag. "It's really so silly. People don't want to lose a dollar's worth of food, so they'll take leftovers home from a restaurant and give them to the kids," Dr. Meyers says. Doing so, he adds, might unknowingly lead to food poisoning.

If you do take home leftovers from dining out, be wise: Refrigerate them as soon as possible and reheat thoroughly before digging in.

Scrub your utensils. Washing utensils in hot water after they've touched raw meat kills offending bacteria.

"A lot of people will cut up their chicken, then cut up their vegetables with the same knife," Garrity says. "They should wash the knife and the cutting board after each use."

Another trap: Using the same utensils to handle raw and cooked meat. If you spear raw meat with a fork, then use the same fork later to serve the meat, you may be transferring bacteria from the raw to the cooked food.

One solution is to cut and prepare the raw meat, then wash your cutting board and utensils in hot, soapy water immediately afterward—before you wash, slice or handle the cooked meat.

Another alternative: Make one cutting board and one cutting knife and fork your designated "before cooking" utensils. Use a second cutting board and any other utensils for the "after." Then you can wash up everything at once, after you're done with food preparation.

DIVERTICULOSIS: PAMPERING YOUR PESKY POUCHES

Question: What do your large intestine and your hair have in common?

Answer: Neither is immune to Father Time.

But while graying hair is obvious, the changes inside your large intestine are not. As you get older, your large intestine is likely to develop small bubblelike pouches called diverticula. The result: a harmless condition called diverticulosis.

"Diverticulosis is not a disease, it's just a phenomenon," says Johns Hopkins' Dr. Schuster. "The diverticula are like hemorrhoids and gray hair—the older you are, the more likely you are to get them."

Up to 20 percent of all people over 50 develop diverticula, doctors say. This is no big problem—except that about 20 percent of those who have diverticulosis can also get diverticulitis, an infection of the diverticula.

"The infection can lead to minute bleeding, abscess or perforation of the colon," Dr. Schuster says. That's why it's important to let your doctor know if you see blood in your stool—particularly if it's dark-colored.

Doctors don't know exactly what causes diverticula, but some experts theorize they form when high pressure in the large intestine pushes against weak spots in the intestinal wall. The high pressure can come from straining during bowel movements or from muscle spasms. Since the intestinal wall weakens with age, the pressure is more likely to cause diverticula when we get older. But doctors also think our low-fiber, high-fat diet boosts our chances of developing diverticula.

Although you can't get rid of diverticula once they've developed, you can prevent them from ever forming. And you can prevent new ones if you do have some.

For diverticula-dousing, fiber is the weapon of choice, says Dr. Meyers. High-fiber foods will keep the pressure off your large intestine, preventing diverticula from popping out. They'll also prevent diverticulitis.

"The fiber keeps things flowing so you don't get infected," Dr. Meyers says. If you stick to the suggested 20 to 35 grams of fiber a day, you have a much lower risk of getting diverticulitis, even if you have diverticulosis. (For tips on boosting your fiber, see "The Ins and Outs of Fiber" on page 68.)

PASSING ON THE GAS

It's not a dinner-table topic, but let's face it, everybody gets gas once in a while. When you do, it's generally for one of two reasons: Either you've swallowed too much air or your body can't completely break down something you've eaten. (Sometimes, although less often, people get gas from a condition called bacterial overgrowth. This occurs when bacteria grow in excess in the small bowel or after certain types of intestinal surgery.)

"When your body can't break down your food, what's not absorbed by the intestines will ferment like wine and make gas," Dr. Meyers says. "But most of the time, you get it from swallowing too much air."

If you have persistent gas, sharp pains or other symptoms, see your doctor. Gas pain that just won't go away might be a symptom of a larger problem, such as lactose intolerance.

"Otherwise, gas is perfectly healthy, even though people are embarrassed by it," Dr. Meyers says.

But here are some food tips to help you control the octane and avoid the embarrassments.

Have your beans and broccoli with charcoal. Certain foods are harder for the body to break down than others because they contain a lot of indigestible fiber. Common gas-producing foods include beans, broccoli, cauliflower, brussels sprouts, cabbage and bran.

But these foods are fiber-filled and healthful. Rather than avoid them, you might want to accompany them with one of grandma's home remedies—charcoal tablets.

Charcoal tablets absorb gas in your gut like a sponge absorbs water, according to Dr. Meyers, who recalls hearing this advice from his grandmother. The saturated charcoal is excreted in your stool without a murmur of gas emission.

Outguess your beans. To minimize the famous after-effects of beans, be sure to soak them for four to five hours before cooking, following the directions in "Cooking without Gas" on page 9. Or try a drop or two of Beano as you're downing your first bite of beans. An enzyme product that aids in digestion and reduces gas, Beano works well with almost any kind of high-fiber food.

Keep a dairy diary. Since many people can't digest dairy foods, their bodies react by producing gas. Record when you eat dairy foods to see if they're related to your gas output. If you go on a nondairy diet for a week or two and have little or no flatulence during that period, you'll know you're on to something.

GALLSTONES: ROLL OUT THE PREVENTION

A rolling stone may gather no moss, but when one of these nasty nodules is hidden in your gallbladder, it'll definitely gather your undivided attention.

"Gallstones give you an aching pain that can go into the chest or even into the right shoulder," says Dr. Miner of the University of Kansas Medical Center. "There's also sometimes a feeling of gas."

Gallstones are usually solidified cholesterol. Some are as tiny as grains of sand, but surgeons have taken out gallstones as large as golf balls. One person can have anywhere from one to several thousand at a time.

Women are more likely than men to have gallstones, and both sexes are more susceptible after the age of 60. Also, Mexicans and Native Americans are more prone to have gallstones than other groups.

A change of diet can't rid you of gallstones. But by making a few changes in your menu, you can help prevent your gallbladder from becoming a stone quarry.

To help save your gallbladder from some rough work, doctors recommend choosing foods that are high in fiber and low in cholesterol (which goes into the formation of gallstones). With a low-cholesterol, high-fiber diet, you're also more likely to keep your weight under control, which is another factor in your favor. "People who are overweight are more susceptible to gallstones," Dr. Miner says.

CELIAC DISEASE: BOOTIN' THE GLUTEN

It's fun to break bread with friends, but when you have celiac disease, bread is more likely to feed regret than friendship.

Also called sprue, celiac disease is a digestive disorder that makes your immune system respond abnormally to gluten, a protein in grains. Immune cells respond to gluten as if it were an invader, causing inflammation and a flattening of the microscopic finger-like projections called villi on the inside of your small intestine. Result: The villi can't absorb food, and your body becomes deficient in many nutrients. People with celiac disease may have stomach cramps and bouts of diarrhea.

There's no cure for celiac disease, but it can be treated very successfully by avoiding gluten altogether. Results from gluten abstention can be dramatic, and you may notice improvement in just a few weeks. Here's how to give gluten the boot.

Go against the grain. Gluten is found primarily in wheat, rye, barley, buckwheat and some oat products. By avoiding foods that contain these grains, especially bread and baked goods, you'll spare your stomach the blues.

Doctors emphasize that it's not difficult to avoid gluten. You're still allowed rice and corn, so you can have rice for your starch, as well as cornbread and rice cakes, plus all the meat, eggs and dairy foods you want.

Watch for gluten incognito. Some innocuous-looking foods may harbor gluten in disguise. Read labels and look for these key terms, since they may signal hidden gluten: stabilizers, emulsifiers, hydrolyzed vegetable or plant protein, or flour that's labeled "unspecified" (which means it comes from an unknown source).

Foods that have these ingredients can include ice cream and frozen yogurt, dips and spreads, chocolate and chocolate products, canned soups, soup mixes and bouillon cubes, lunch meats and condiments. And be cautious with mustard and ketchup, since some brands also contain gluten.

Seek a network safety net. The national Celiac Sprue Association provides advice and information to anyone who has this problem. If your doctor says you have celiac disease, be sure to ask for the current address or telephone number of the association.

LACTOSE INTOLERANCE: AVOIDING UDDER PRODUCTS

Most people develop lactose intolerance naturally when their bodies stop producing enough lact*ase*, an enzyme that breaks down lact*ose*, the sugar that is found in milk and dairy products. When this happens, the food just lazes around your intestines like fermenting wine in a wine keg, says Johns Hopkins' Dr. Schuster.

"We tend to think of lactose intolerance as the exception to the rule, but the only people who seem to be lactose *tolerant* are in Europe or in European-based cultures like ours," says Dennis A. Savaiano, Ph.D., associate dean and professor of food science and nutrition at the University of Minnesota College of Human Ecology in St. Paul.

Approximately 75 percent of African Americans, Jews, Native Americans and Hispanics are lactose intolerant to some degree, as are 90 percent of Asian Americans. Symptoms include nausea, cramps, bloating, gas and diarrhea that begin 30 minutes to two hours after dairy foods are eaten.

Here's how to detour the dairy aisle and live without lactose.

Denounce dairy. The Cleveland Clinic's Dr. Ruderman suggests approaching the following dairy foods with caution: milk, ice cream, cream soups and soft cheeses. "A large number of digestive complaints can be stopped just by avoiding milk and milk products," he says.

But don't be fooled by low-fat or skim milk, which is just as risky as regular milk. Nearly all kinds of milk contain 12 to 13 grams of lactose in each eight-ounce serving.

Try yogurt for an exception. Even though yogurt has almost as much lactose as milk, the bacteria in yogurt—the so-called live cultures—naturally break down lactose in the intestine and counter the symptoms in people who are lactose intolerant.

One study by the Department of Food Science and Nutrition at the University of Minnesota in St. Paul supports this advice. In a study of ten lactose-intolerant men and women, researchers found they did a better job of digesting the lactose in yogurt than the lactose in any other dairy food.

Mimic milk. If you can't put Elsie and her products out to pasture, Mount Sinai's Dr. Meyers suggests trying low-lactose milk or ice cream. For example, Lactaid, one widely available brand of low-lactose milk, has 8 grams or less of lactose, compared with the 12 to 13 grams in milk. "Low-lactose milk will sometimes do the trick for some people, especially if they just want to put a little in their coffee," Dr. Meyers says.

Lactaid also comes in tablets, which you can take before eating dairy products, and in drops, which you add to milk. Both of these help break down lactose, making it easy to digest.

HOW TO EVADE LURKING LACTOSE

A very small proportion of people who are lactose intolerant are extremely sensitive to lactose.

If you're among them, avoiding lactose may be a lot harder than just shunning the milk aisle. When you read labels, be on the lookout for the words *whey, curds, milk by-products, dry milk solids* and *nonfat dry milk powder*. And of course, avoid any food that has milk or lactose listed on the label.

Here are some surprising foods that may be surreptitious sources of lactose.

- Breads and baked goods.
- Processed cereals and mixes for pancakes, cookies and biscuits.
- Instant potatoes and soups.
- Breakfast drinks.
- Nonkosher lunch meats.
- Salad dressings.
- Candies.
- Nondairy products such as coffee creamers and whipped toppings.

Doctors emphasize, however, that sensitivity to these foods is rare. "Anyone this sensitive should see a physician to find out if there is a complicating factor or another cause for the lactose intolerance," says Dr. Dennis Savaiano of the University of Minnesota College of Human Ecology.

TRAVELER'S DIARRHEA: COME HOME WITHOUT IT

Traveling can indeed be educational. But if you've ever encountered traveler's diarrhea in your globetrotting, you may have learned a travel lesson that will last a lifetime.

Diarrhea can strike anywhere, of course, and can be caused by many factors, including bacterial infection and poor food absorption or digestion. Among infections, one of the meanest banditos is caused by *Giardia*, a common water- and foodborne organism that can cause profuse diarrhea.

Getting diarrhea can do more than just ruin your plans and leave you feeling battered. It can drain your body of fluids that contain vital minerals and nutrients, Dr. Ruderman warns. So not only do you need to battle the bug, you also have to find a way to get some fluids into your system as soon as possible.

When in Rome, don't do as the Romans do. A dream vacation can quickly turn into a nightmare if you drink and dine like the natives. To be safe, always peel your fruit and drink bottled beverages. Don't even rinse with tapwater when you brush your teeth, Dr. Meyers cautions.

Help your rehydration with sugar. After a bad bout of diarrhea, you've lost a lot of water—but sugary foods may help you get rehydrated. That's because sugar helps your body retain liquid.

To increase fluid quickly, try drinking defizzed regular soda. (Diet soda won't do the trick because it's so low in sugar.) Better yet, make this rehydration drink recommended by the World Health Organization: In a liter of water (a little more than a quart),

FOR THE TROUBLED TUMMY, WET YOUR WHISTLE

Stomach troubles that lead to diarrhea or excessive vomiting can deplete your body of vital fluids, so it's important to put back what nature takes away.

The first source to tap is the nearest one: water. But while water replaces lost liquids, it doesn't replenish vitamins. Also, water doesn't do anything to replace essential electrolytes—chemicals like sodium, potassium, calcium and magnesium that the body needs to function normally. Commercial sports drinks are better, since they contain vitamins and minerals. And there are many nutrient-rich beverages that you can buy or concoct to rev up your depleted system.

Be selective about fruit juices, however. One study in the Netherlands found that of 17 children and 12 adults given apple juice, 7 of the children did not thoroughly digest the fructose, a type of sugar, in the apple juice. (Only 4 of the adults had problems digesting the fructose.) This poor fructose digestion can cause excessive diarrhea in children, the study concluded.

Pulpy juices such as orange juice, however, may be good because their high fiber content absorbs water and firms up stool.

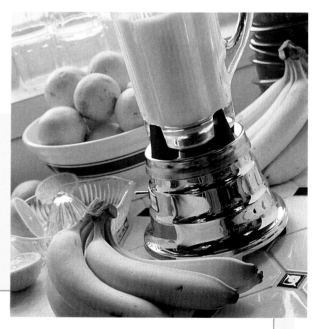

SHAKE THE DEHYDRATION BLUES

Here's an easy and delicious way to replace energy lost during brief bouts of dehydration: Blend one medium-size banana into one eight-ounce serving of orange juice. The orange juice has vital vitamins (mostly C and B's), water and 112 energy-boosting calories. The banana has potassium (451 milligrams), fiber and pectin, which absorb water and help stop diarrhea.

mix ½ teaspoon of table salt, ¼ teaspoon of potassium chloride (found in salt substitutes), ½ teaspoon of baking soda and 4 tablespoons of sugar. Stir until all the ingredients are dissolved, then drink it down. (Of course, if you're in a foreign country when you need this remedy, be sure to use bottled water.)

Top off the tank. In addition to sugary drinks, restock your body with clear liquids such as broth or apple juice. Avoid alcoholic drinks, because alcohol acts like a diuretic, draining more fluids from your kidneys.

BRATs to the rescue. When you're ready to eat solid foods after weathering a bout of diarrhea, try eating *ba*nanas, *r*ice, *a*pplesauce and *t*oast, foods that are least likely to worsen diarrhea. In fact, the fiber they contain helps dry things up.

Try a psyllium solution. Crushed psyllium seeds are an excellent way to stanch the flow of diarrhea, according to Dr. Schuster.

"People think of psyllium as a bulking agent. It loves water and binds with it," Dr. Schuster says.

Psyllium is a primary ingredient in many over-the-counter laxatives, including Metamucil. Take it in powdered form with lots of water. You can also buy psyllium in large bottles at many health food stores.

CONSTIPATION AND HEMORRHOIDS: RESULTS WITHOUT FORCING

Constipation happens. A poor diet can bring it on and so can travel, overuse of laxatives and even stress.

"Constipation is often related to stress," says Dr. Ruderman. "But if after a week or two you see no change in your bowel habits, you should check it out, because it certainly can herald a more serious problem."

And constipation often has a sidekick—hemorrhoids. These occur when veins on the inside of the anus become swollen, just as varicose veins can swell up in your leg.

A RECIPE FOR RELIEF

Your dried-fruit shelf has the fixin's for a laxative to get things moving in the right direction. Although this recipe makes four servings, it's fairly potent and not recommended for daily consumption—so plan on freezing some of it. Eat one serving (about ½ cup) in the morning, then allow for the compote to take effect. Have more the next morning if necessary.

Fruit-Lax

½	cup dried figs
½	cup dried apricots
½	cup prunes
1	pint water
1	pint apricot nectar

Makes 4 servings.

Per serving: 221 calories, 0.6 g. fat (2% of calories), 5.7 g. dietary fiber, 0 mg. cholesterol, 13.2 mg. sodium.

"Hemorrhoids can bulge out, bleed and cause problems," Dr. Ruderman says. Doctors have many techniques for removing them. However, Dr. Ruderman emphasizes, "most hemorrhoids can be treated without surgery, with minor changes in the diet, warm soaks in the tub, attention to hygiene, and sometimes the use of medical suppositories."

For both constipation and hemorrhoid prevention, exercise can help bring relief, because it gets things moving through the intestinal tract. But along with brisk walking, here are some shrewd food moves that will give your bound-up bowels a break.

Fiber up. Fiber helps counter constipation and prevent hemorrhoids. For more information on fiber and ways to get it, see "The Ins and Outs of Fiber" on page 68 and "Target Your Health" on page 69.

Imbibe abundantly. Asking your digestion to work without water is like munching dry crackers in the Sahara. Your digestive tract doesn't like to work without fluids, so drink six to eight eight-ounce glasses of fluids, preferably water, a day. Adding liquid to your body will ease digestion and loosen stool.

CROON FOR PRUNES

There have been many positive reports on prunes and their use as a natural laxative, but even after a lot of study, what causes prunes' potency remains a mystery. Experts think it's something in their chemical makeup.

A pioneering experiment more than 50 years ago by researcher George Emerson at the University of California in San Francisco found that even watered-down prune extract caused contractions in the intestines of rabbits. A later study, similar in design, at Boston University found that prune juice caused more fluid output in humans than other food.

Some researchers have speculated that prunes contain a natural chemical compound that resembles a laxative drug.

Diabetes: How to Lift the Sugar Blues

Carl's Confectionery Company is a large manufacturer of boxed chocolates. Every hour on the hour, Carl's candy machines spit out one million chocolate candies onto a conveyor belt that carries them to Carl's crew of well-trained laborers, who swiftly and skillfully pack the chocolates in boxes.

Suppose half of Carl's chocolate packers fail to show up for work one day. Or maybe the boxes are defective and the workers can't open the lids. But the machines are *still* producing one million chocolates per hour.

The result? Chocolates scattered all over the place. If this continues, Carl will be out of business.

This not-so-sweet scenario is a lot like what happens in your body if you're one of the 14 million Americans with diabetes. Instead of chocolates, however, we're talking about blood sugar, or glucose. Here's what happens.

DANGER: A GLUCOSE GLUT

Our bodies produce glucose from the foods we eat, and our cells convert it into energy. But glucose can't get into cells without the help of insulin. If the pancreas fails to produce enough insulin, or if the insulin isn't good at its job, the glucose has no place to go. Soon the bloodstream is caught in the throes of a glucose glut.

Why is this so bad? Prolonged high blood sugar levels can damage the blood vessels, eyes, nerves and kidneys. Complications can range from impotence and blindness to loss of limbs. In fact, diabetes is the fourth leading cause of death in the United States, costing 160,000 lives every year, says F. Xavier Pi-Sunyer, M.D., director of endocrinology at St. Luke's–Roosevelt Hospital in New York, professor of medicine at Columbia University and past president of the American Diabetes Association (ADA).

The kind of diabetes that affects younger people is called Type I, or insulin-dependent, diabetes, in which the pancreas produces no insulin at all. Fortunately, Type I is uncommon, representing about 10 percent of all cases.

The majority of people with diabetes have Type II, or non-insulin-dependent, diabetes. This type occurs when the pancreas produces some insulin, but not enough to get the job done. Or perhaps the pancreas produces enough of the hormone, but for some reason the body is resistant to its effects.

TURNING THE TABLES ON DIABETES

Diabetes may at first produce only mild symptoms, such as increased hunger and thirst or the need to urinate often. As a result, millions of Americans are walking around with sky-high blood sugar levels without knowing it, says Aaron Vinik, M.D., Ph.D., director of the Diabetes Research Institute in Nor-

INSULIN IN ACTION

Here's how the hormone insulin works in the body when all systems are go.

After you eat, levels of an energy-producing sugar called glucose rise in the bloodstream. The pancreas responds by secreting insulin, which helps the blood sugar enter into individual cells.

Diabetes occurs when this system somehow breaks down. If the pancreas doesn't produce enough insulin, or if the body has trouble using it efficiently, blood sugar levels can go sky-high—a condition called hyperglycemia—and that can have adverse effects on many organs and body functions.

folk, Virginia. "They only become aware that their health is in danger after a blood test from a routine physical exam reveals they have diabetes." That's why everyone over 40, especially if they are overweight or have a family history of the disease, should have their blood tested once a year.

"For a great number of people, poor eating habits and a sedentary lifestyle seem to trigger the gene that causes Type II diabetes," says Dr. Vinik. He urges people who are at risk to make positive lifestyle changes, which can dramatically reduce their chances of developing the disease in the first place.

For starters, get plenty of exercise. Every time you take a brisk walk or ride an exercise bicycle, you burn up much of the glucose accumulating in your bloodstream, says Dr. Vinik. In addition, exercise helps make cells less resistant to insulin.

The second and perhaps most important lifestyle adjustment is to pay close attention to what you eat. That means watching your weight and keeping an eye on your daily menu.

TIPPING THE SCALES IN YOUR FAVOR

About 85 percent of people with Type II diabetes are overweight, researchers say. Further, when overweight verges on obesity, health risks *really* shoot up. Although the pancreas works overtime when you're overweight, it just can't produce enough insulin. At the same time, extra weight makes the cells more resistant to the insulin that is produced.

"If you have a family history of diabetes but keep your weight under control, there's a good chance you may never even get it," says Stanley Mirsky, M.D., associate clinical professor of metabolic diseases at Mount Sinai School of Medicine in New York and author of *Controlling Diabetes the Easy Way.* "And in those who do have it, even a slight weight loss of five to ten pounds may be all it takes to keep blood glucose levels within normal limits."

THE STRAIGHT SCOOP ON SUGAR

Many people think that diabetes is strictly a problem of sugar consumption. But it's not that simple. "There is

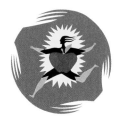

BREAKTHROUGHS IN HEALING

1 9 2 1

Frederick Banting and Charles Best extract insulin from a dog pancreas and discover that it lowers blood sugar levels in dogs. One year later, they duplicate their findings with humans.

1 9 8 7

Noted fiber researcher James W. Anderson, M.D., demonstrates the effectiveness of high-fiber diets in controlling blood sugar levels and reducing insulin requirements.

1 9 9 3

The Diabetes Control Complications Trial, a ten-year nationwide study, concludes that improved blood sugar control significantly lowers an individual's risk of developing all blood complications.

1 9 9 4

The American Diabetes Association publishes dietary guidelines advocating an individualized approach. The guidelines recommend daily consumption of 20 to 35 grams of dietary fiber from a wide variety of food sources and consumption of carbohydrates based on individual treatment goals.

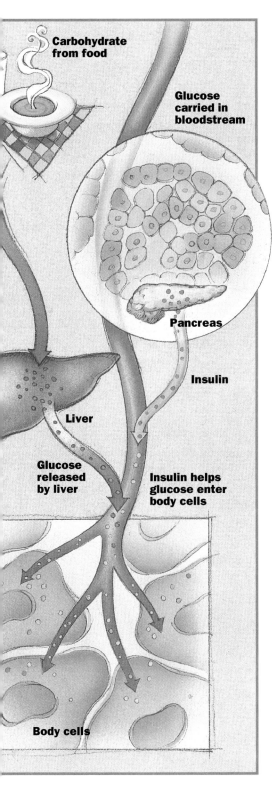

Carbohydrate from food

Glucose carried in bloodstream

Pancreas

Insulin

Liver

Glucose released by liver

Insulin helps glucose enter body cells

Body cells

Back to Basics, Hawaiian-Style

The link between diet and diabetes is very strong, if native Hawaiians are any indication. "Generations ago, Hawaiians were rarely fat," observes Terry Shintani, M.D., director of preventive medicine at the Waianae Coast Comprehensive Health Center. "It's only since the introduction of the typical American-style diet to the islands that we have seen such a dramatic incidence of obesity and obesity-related diseases such as diabetes."

Dr. Shintani and a growing number of other researchers think islanders will be healthier if they return to their native diet. At his clinic, Dr. Shintani has put a number of patients on a diet of taro (a starchy native root), poi, seaweed, sweet potatoes, greens, fruit and fish—all foods native to the island. Such a diet is low in fat, high in fiber and complex carbohydrates and has a moderate amount of protein.

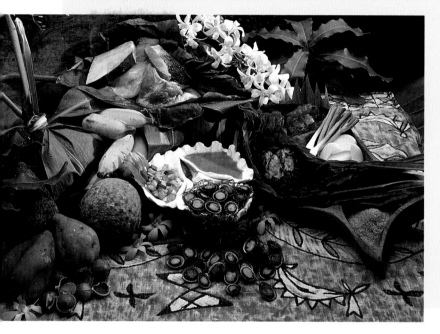

The results of switching to this traditional Hawaiian fare have been fantastic, according to Dr. Shintani. One patient taking insulin for her diabetes, for example, was able to go off insulin entirely.

Native Hawaiian fresh foods—including fish, shellfish, fresh fruits and vegetables—helped keep diabetes in check.

little scientific evidence that sugar is any more dangerous for people with diabetes than it is for people without it," says Marion Franz, R.D., director of nutrition and publications at the International Diabetes Center in Minneapolis.

That's great news for people who think that diabetes means saying sayonara to sweets. But we shouldn't accept that news as permission to go hog-wild with the sweet stuff.

Too much sugar at one time can cause a sudden and dramatic surge in blood glucose levels. This surge can be caused by sugar in any form, including numerous kinds of sweeteners such as corn syrup, fruit juice and honey. So keep the following sugar guidelines in mind.

Grab some fruit. You can eat fruit without raising blood sugar levels very significantly, according to Franz. When you crave something sweet, reach for an apple, orange or banana, she says.

Avoid fruit drinks and juices. When you drink fruit juices, you're getting a high-octane dose of sugar. So instead of swigging a big glass of OJ at breakfast, you may be better off eating whole fruit.

Watch out for cover-ups. Are you eating more sugar than you think? One way to find out is by reading package labels; the sugar content of many packaged and processed foods is surprisingly high. Sugar sometimes goes by different names, such as sucrose, fructose and sorbitol. If you find any of these ranked at the top of the ingredient list, the label is telling you the food product has a lot of sugar. *Note:* You can't always assume that foods promoted "for diabetics" are recommended by doctors or approved by the ADA. In fact, the ADA discourages food manufacturers from promoting any particular food in this way. So always be sure to read the ingredient list and consider how any food fits into your total diet.

Go for sugar substitutes. Aspartame (NutraSweet) has far fewer calories than sugar, and saccharin has none. Neither raises blood sugar levels at all, so they're safe and smart alternatives.

THE TAKE-CHARGE APPROACH

To effectively control diabetes, you need to unlearn a lifetime of eating habits and adopt a new, very targeted approach to eating. For many, the key to losing weight, controlling blood sugar levels and preventing diabetes complications is as simple as following a few basic dietary guidelines.

Be a linguine lover. Most of the glucose in our bloodstream comes either from simple carbohydrates (better known as sugars) or from complex carbohydrates (better known as starches).

In the past, the ADA guidelines specified the percentages of complex carbohydrates that should be included in the diet. The current guidelines say the amount should depend on individual needs. As a general rule, however, Dr. Vinik suggests that 50 to 60 percent of your calories should come from carbohydrates. Good sources of complex carbs include pasta, bread, potatoes and whole grains.

Trim the fat. Not only are fatty foods, well, fattening, they also tend to make insulin less effective.

Even a little fat in the diet can be a problem. Just an extra 40 grams of fat per day (roughly equal to a quarter-pound burger with large fries) may triple your risk for Type II diabetes, according to a study at the University of Colorado Health Sciences Center in Denver.

While individual recommendations vary, and you should discuss your diet with your physician. Most doctors recommend that people with diabetes monitor the amount of total calories that come from fat. (As a general rule, many experts say you should aim for 25 percent of total calories from fat—and if you have diabetes, your own

doctor may recommend much less.)

Go easy on protein. Yes, you need some protein. But too much can significantly increase your chances of developing kidney complications—which are an added risk for people with diabetes, says Dr. Vinik. Try to reduce your consumption of protein to somewhere between 10 and 15 percent of total calories. For most people, that's the equivalent of two glasses of skim milk and a serving of lean meat per day.

Favor some fiber. A high-fiber diet—essential for weight loss and digestive health—is also helpful for those with diabetes.

Some studies have shown that a diet rich in fiber will indirectly lower blood sugar levels by slowing the rate at which food is converted into glucose and absorbed into the bloodstream, says New York endocrinologist Dr. Pi-Sunyer. Foods that are high in fiber include beans, corn, oat bran and fruit.

Most people should eat 20 to 35 grams of total fiber a day, according to Dr. Pi-Sunyer. As you get used to meals that are high in fiber, you can actually eat even more, he says.

Become a grazer. Eating too much starch at one time can send blood sugar into orbit, says Dr. Mirsky. For this reason, many experts recommend that you spread your calorie consumption throughout the day. But be careful that you don't eat more just because you're eating more frequently.

Bag the booze. Not only is alcohol fattening, it also can aggravate damage to nerves or the liver brought on by diabetes, says Dr. Vinik. He recommends drinking no more than 8 ounces of wine or 24 ounces of beer per week.

NUTRIENTS YOU CAN COUNT ON

Not getting enough essential nutrients can cause blood sugar levels to rise and increase the risk of developing complications such as nerve and kidney damage, says Dr. Mirsky.

In addition to eating a proper diet,

Chrome-Plated Protection

A growing body of evidence suggests that a great way to prevent Type II diabetes, as well as its complications, is to get more chromium in the diet.

As we get older, blood sugar and insulin levels commonly rise as insulin's ability to metabolize sugar diminishes. This results in a condition called glucose intolerance, which is an early precursor of full-blown diabetes.

Some researchers blame this on the fact that most of us don't get enough chromium in our diet. Adding chromium seems to make insulin more efficient and improves its ability to control blood sugar, says Richard A. Anderson, Ph.D., a biochemist with the U.S. Department of Agriculture Human Nutrition Research Center in Beltsville, Maryland.

In one study, Dr. Anderson looked at 17 patients, 8 with mild glucose intolerance and 9 without. For five weeks, he gave them 200 micrograms of chromium. Those with normal glucose tolerance experienced no changes. But the glucose-intolerant group saw their blood sugar levels fall as much as 50 percent.

"A significant number of the people we see with elevated blood glucose have low chromium intake," says Dr. Anderson. "But blood glucose levels normalize in 80 to 90 percent of the people to whom we give additional chromium. We speculate that adequate chromium intake could prevent many cases of mild glucose intolerance from progressing to Type II diabetes."

Chromium may also play an important role in fighting diabetes-related heart disease. It does this by favorably altering blood cholesterol levels. "When insulin levels rise, plaque formation increases in the arteries, raising your risk for heart disease," observes Dr. Anderson. "By making insulin more effective, you need less, so plaque formation may be hindered."

Chromium is a trace mineral. This means there's less of it in our diet than magnesium or calcium.

Good dietary sources of chromium include brans, whole-grain cereals and breads, barley, brewer's yeast, liver and other organ meats, turkey ham, green beans, broccoli, grape juice and various fruits.

The research isn't all in, but some doctors believe that chromium deficiencies are very common. "Ninety percent of our diets are marginally deficient in chromium," says Dr. Anderson. He recommends we take chromium supplements to the tune of 200 micrograms per day for maximum protection. (That's well within the limits for safe intake.) Also, Dr. Anderson recommends we keep in mind these chromium facts.

■ High intakes of simple sugars and sugary foods will cause you to excrete chromium.

■ Complex carbohydrates like pasta and potatoes tend to help the body hold onto its chromium reserves.

■ Stress and anxiety deplete our chromium reserves.

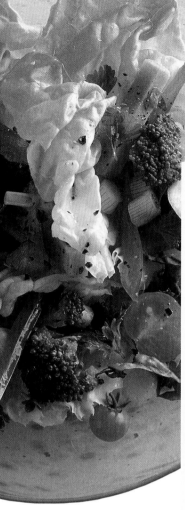

BROCCOLI AND TURKEY HAM SALAD

Here's a tasty way to make sure that you're getting a healthy dose of diabetes-fighting chromium—a chromium-packed tossed salad! Each serving has 27 micrograms of the nutrient.

4	**cups small broccoli florets**
1	**sweet red pepper, cut into thin strips**
2	**stalks celery, thinly sliced**
4	**ounces turkey ham, cut into thin strips**
¼	**cup finely chopped scallions**
2	**tablespoons defatted chicken stock**
1	**tablespoon olive oil**
1	**tablespoon lemon juice**
½	**teaspoon ground black pepper**
¼	**teaspoon dried basil**
1	**small head Boston lettuce**
8	**cherry tomatoes, halved**
2	**tablespoons fresh parsley leaves**
4	**whole-wheat rolls**

Steam the broccoli for 4 minutes, or until just crisp-tender. Place in a large bowl and let cool for 10 minutes. Add the red peppers, celery, turkey ham and scallions. Toss lightly.

In a small bowl, whisk together the stock, oil, lemon juice, black pepper and basil. Pour over the broccoli mixture and toss to mix well.

Divide the head of lettuce into individual leaves and use to line dinner plates. Top with the broccoli mixture and garnish with the tomatoes and parsley. Serve with the rolls.

Makes 4 servings.

Per serving: 198 calories, 6.1 g. fat (25% of calories), 6 g. dietary fiber, 18 mg. cholesterol, 547 mg. sodium.

Chromium deficiencies are very common, but they needn't be. This trace mineral is found in such common foods as broccoli, whole grains and a variety of fruits.

many people may need to take a daily multivitamin, Dr. Mirsky says. Among the vitamins and minerals you need if you have diabetes, here are the leaders.

Boost your biotin. Many people with Type II diabetes have significantly lower concentrations of the B vitamin biotin in their bodies. One Japanese study found that taking a nine-milligram supplement of biotin daily corrected high blood sugar levels in 43 people who had Type II diabetes. You'll find a heaping helping of biotin in such foods as milk, vegetables, nuts, whole grains and tuna.

Go for the B_6. Vitamin B_6 has been shown to control high blood sugar levels in pregnant women, says Dr. Mirsky. A diet rich in B_6 has also been used to treat diabetes-related nerve damage. Meats, fish, beans, poultry, grains and green leafy vegetables all contain generous amounts of this important vitamin.

But don't take B_6 supplements without a doctor's supervision, since it can be toxic at high doses.

Lift your magnesium. Experts observe that magnesium deficiencies make our cells resistant to insulin and contribute to atherosclerosis and high blood pressure. You can get plenty of magnesium from foods such as green vegetables, beans, nuts and grains.

HYPOGLYCEMIA: THE BOOMERANG EFFECT

Sometimes diabetes can make a U-turn and actually send blood sugar levels plunging rather than rising. This condition is called hypoglycemia, and it can produce such frightening symptoms as dizziness, tremors, weakness, sweating and headache. What makes blood sugar levels flip-flop? "We usually see it when patients overexercise, go on crash diets or take extra-high doses of insulin," says Dr. Vinik.

"These people lose sight of the goal of diabetes management, which is to achieve a normal blood glucose level," Dr. Vinik adds. "And that can only be achieved through normal exercise and maintaining a normal weight."

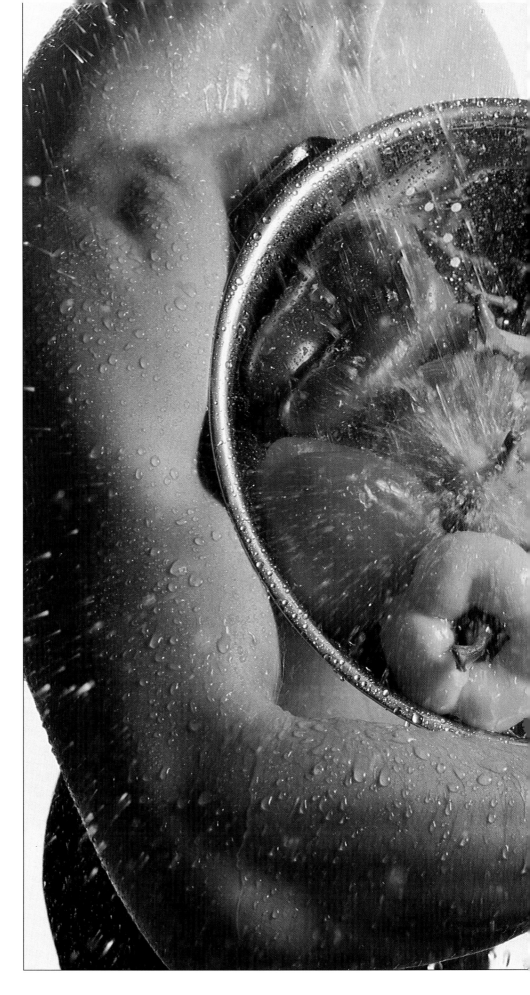

PART THREE

High-Power Nutrition for Cellular Health

Every cell

needs help

to battle

the body's

invaders

Y our body is a beehive of activity—with swarms of defenders to guard your cells. These include millions of killer T-cells, antibodies, macrophages and other infection-fighters, all armed against hostile takeovers.

But even these swarms of cellular bodyguards can't totally guard your body from the cost of time. Age takes its toll on your cells. Some get damaged. Others become battle-worn. The ongoing routine of renovation and replacement begins to slow down.

Today, scientists have discovered a great deal about the processes that cause greatest damage to our cells—including aging, infections and disease. They are beginning to understand which nutrients the cells need and which cell intruders cause the most damage. They have begun to understand which cancer-causing agents can make cell reproduction run amok. They've learned volumes about the body's guardians—killer T-cells and their cousins—that glide through the system and stop disease-causing invaders in their tracks.

Best of all, research has now made a direct link between some of the foods we eat and the power of those foods to help protect our cells from all attackers. The result: new insights that can help us change our diets so we can live longer, feel healthier and help ward off a host of life-threatening diseases.

CHAPTER SEVEN

Rejuvenate Your Body with "Youth Foods"

The building looked almost brand new until someone came along with a wrecking ball.

At first when the ball started swinging, you didn't see much damage. A window smashed here. A cornice there. A small hole in the roof. Still, how much of this battering could the building take?

Then something peculiar started to happen. After a couple of days of steady pounding, the wrecking ball was doing less damage. It kept swinging away, but now it bounced more often than it landed.

The building, it now appeared, would be safe and sound for a long, long time.

CRASHERS AT THE CELL GATES

Until recently, researchers didn't understand much about the cellular wrecking balls that threaten good health and youthful living—the darting, antagonistic, submicroscopic cell-wall invaders called free radicals.

Free radicals are really just highly reactive molecules roaming in search of a partner. These wrecking-ball marauders aren't alive, but the way they damage cells certainly affects *our* lives. What makes them so interactive is a purely chemical reaction. That reaction—known as the oxidation process—sets free radicals loose inside our innocent cells.

"You can't pinpoint free radicals because they are fleeting, and they react so quickly with anything they come in con-

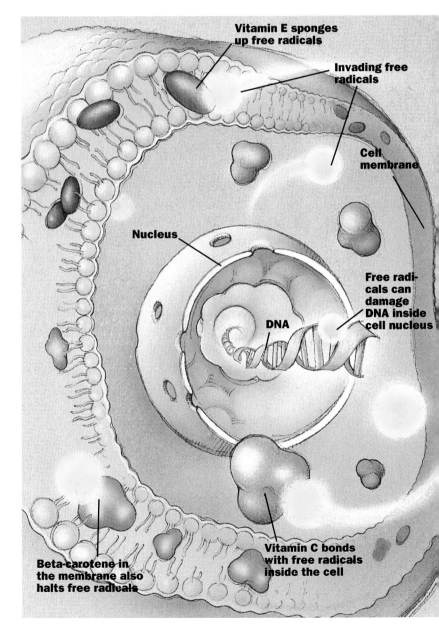

Vitamin E sponges up free radicals

Invading free radicals

Cell membrane

Nucleus

Free radicals can damage DNA inside cell nucleus

DNA

Beta-carotene in the membrane also halts free radicals

Vitamin C bonds with free radicals inside the cell

tact with," notes Pamela Starke-Reed, Ph.D., director of the Office of Nutrition at the National Institute on Aging (NIA). "You can't create the reaction in a lab and say, a-ha, see that little speck there? That's a free radical. But you can look at a nick in the DNA chain or a break in the cell membrane and see the results of free radical damage."

TOP DEFENDERS

On the other side, protecting our bodies from the onslaught of these gate crashers, are chemicals and nutrients identified as antioxidants. Some antioxidants occur naturally in our cells; others

RAIDERS IN SEARCH OF LOST ELECTRONS

"We have met the enemy and he is us," said Pogo, the savviest of all comic-strip characters. He might have been talking about free radicals—roving gangs of oxygen molecules in the blood that mug (oxidize) our aging cells, causing disease and early decay.

Free radicals are by-products of normal metabolism, produced in enormous numbers by stresses such as air pollution, x-rays, injuries—and aging itself. They first slide into delinquency when they lose an electron while burning fuel. To replace it, they raid molecules in neighboring cells, which are then initiated into the gang. Sacrificing an electron, they become new free radicals.

Like particles of rust on a piece of iron, free radicals multiply in every cell by the tens of thousands every day. Under normal conditions, however, your body can neutralize the threat. Your own natural enzymes disarm free radicals with the help of antioxidant nutrients. Vitamin E and vitamin A (from beta-carotene) absorb radicals before they can damage outer cell membranes. And vitamin C bonds with radicals in the liquid inside cells, which is eventually drawn out and flushed away into the urine.

can be found in some foods.

So how do scientists know that dietary antioxidants are really free radical busters?

By looking at what's *not* visible, Dr. Starke-Reed says. "In the presence of antioxidants, what you do see is much less free radical damage occurring."

As for the reaction itself, it's happening all the time in nature. Leave a stick of margarine on the shelf during a warm summer day, and soon you'll catch the odor of a free radical free-for-all. In fact, the process of cell decay is like margarine going rancid, according to Mohsen Meydani, Ph.D., associate professor of nutrition at Tufts University in Boston and a researcher at the U.S. Department of Agriculture (USDA) Human Nutrition Research Center on Aging at the university. Like the fat in margarine, the fats within our cells start to decay—or oxidize—when oxygen reaches them.

"That's how skin wrinkles, the body weakens and muscles lose their youthful tone," Dr. Meydani says. As these changes occur at the cellular level, the immune cells in our bodies also can lose their ability to function. "That's also why older people are more susceptible to infection," he adds.

Your body has defenses, however—built-in enzyme forces that normally keep free radicals at controllable levels. Enzymes are protein molecules that speed up chemical reactions in cells. Without their protection, our bodies would literally spoil at top speed, making us old before our time.

Three of these enzymes work as antioxidants. Through a complex chemical process, the enzymes channel the energies of excess free radicals into harmless substances like water and ordinary oxygen.

Our bodies usually respond to the presence of increased free radicals by boosting production of the antioxidant enzymes. Trained athletes, for example, have higher levels of antioxidant enzymes than the rest of us. That's how their bodies adapt to the extra free radicals produced by strenuous exercise.

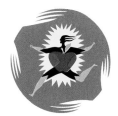

BREAKTHROUGHS IN HEALING

1945

Physician brothers E. V. and Wilfred Shute first use vitamin E to treat heart disease. Their second patient is E. V.'s barber, who appears to be dying. Three weeks after vitamin E is injected, he's playing tympani in the local theater.

1954

The free radical theory of aging is first put forth by Denham Harmon, M.D., Ph.D. His research suggests that chemical compounds that fight free radicals might slow aging.

1991

A report from the Gerontology Research Center at the National Institute on Aging in Baltimore concludes that antioxidants may be important in determining the frequency of diseases that are related to aging.

1992–93

In a Harvard-associated Nurses Health Study of 87,000 women, researchers find that those who eat 15 to 20 milligrams a day of beta-carotene and of vitamin E have 40 percent fewer heart attacks and strokes than women who consumed less than 6 milligrams a day.

But since most of us don't have these extra reserves, our cells need all the help they can get in order to face free radical assaults. Especially damaging are everyday toxins and pollutants like first- and second-hand cigarette smoke, car exhaust fumes and other infamous health wreckers.

THE CRUNCHY FOUNTAIN OF YOUTH

While you can't spend your life dodging pollutants, what you can do is rebuild your natural antioxidant defenses. And a lot of that rebuilding can be done by being selective about the foods you eat.

Since antioxidant nutrients are not made in the body like the enzymes, they need to be replenished every day. And that's where a high-antioxidant diet comes in.

Researchers are convinced that three of the most potent and valuable antioxidants are vitamin C, vitamin E and beta-carotene. In a review conducted by the Gerontology Research Center of the National Institute on Aging in Baltimore, researchers concluded that antioxidant levels in our bodies may help determine how many age-related diseases we have, as well as the general status of our health.

Fortunately, we don't have to look very far to find these antioxidants. Many fruits and vegetables are loaded with them.

But to get adequate amounts of antioxidant protection from your diet, researchers agree that you need to be truly diligent about eating no fewer than five servings of fruits and vegetables every day. Unfortunately, fewer than 10 percent of Americans get this daily dose of defense.

What happens if you do eat lots of flavorful fruits and tender-crisp vegetables? Not only do they give you plenty of day-in, day-out, rejuvenating antioxidants, but these foods have a bonus, too. They are natural sources of fiber, which helps

THE BETA-CAROTENE BULL'S-EYE

Beta-carotene is an important youth-preserving antioxidant, and just a single daily serving of fruits or vegetables rich in this nutrient may also reduce your risk of heart attack and stroke. In the target below, the best sources are nearest to the bull's-eye.

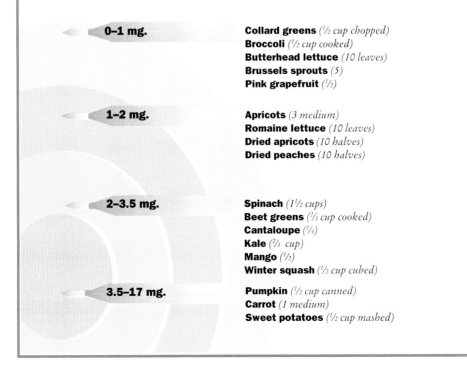

0–1 mg.

Collard greens (*½ cup chopped*)
Broccoli (*½ cup cooked*)
Butterhead lettuce (*10 leaves*)
Brussels sprouts (*5*)
Pink grapefruit (*½*)

1–2 mg.

Apricots (*3 medium*)
Romaine lettuce (*10 leaves*)
Dried apricots (*10 halves*)
Dried peaches (*10 halves*)

2–3.5 mg.

Spinach (*1½ cups*)
Beet greens (*⅔ cup cooked*)
Cantaloupe (*¼*)
Kale (*⅔ cup*)
Mango (*½*)
Winter squash (*½ cup cubed*)

3.5–17 mg.

Pumpkin (*½ cup canned*)
Carrot (*1 medium*)
Sweet potatoes (*½ cup mashed*)

CONQUERING CATARACTS

Cataracts cloud the vision of 20 percent of Americans over 65. How to avoid them? Make sure that your diet includes lots of antioxidant-rich fruits and vegetables. Just 3½ servings a day of foods high in antioxidants will make the difference, researchers report. People who eat less are six times more likely to get cataracts as they age, studies show.

Scientists believe that antioxidant vitamins like C and E prevent oxidation of proteins in the lens of the eye, which may lead to cataracts. And although beta-carotene doesn't reach the lens, you should eat your carrots anyway. Orange-yellow veggies are also full of other carotenoid antioxidants, such as alpha-carotene, lycopene and cryptoxanthan, that do penetrate and defend the lens.

Carrots, grapefruit, cantaloupe and lettuce—along with other dark green, leafy vegetables—are all sources of eye-protecting carotenoids.

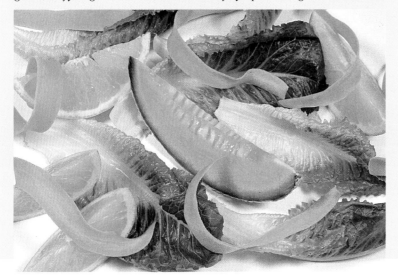

keep cholesterol at bay and your digestive system in tune. Round out your meals with protein, calcium and zinc—from whole grains, low-fat dairy products and small quantities of lean meat—and you're on your way to a longer, healthier life.

Here's a closer look at the true youth foods.

BETAS YOU CAN BET ON

Rabbit food comes from a family that's almost as large as, well, a family of rabbits. Beta-carotene, one of the star achievers in the crowd of compounds known as carotenoids, has more than 500 related compounds. Their chemical structure gives them an orange-yellow pigment that stands out on the produce shelf like a full-color ad for good health. But dark green vegetables are also great sources of these compounds (as well as other antioxidants), so when you go in search of these youth boosters, you have a lot of choices.

Beta-carotene is one of four related compounds, called carotenes, that are converted to vitamin A in the body. It is the most common carotene in the human food supply, says Robert Russell, M.D., a researcher at the USDA Human Nutrition Research Center at Tufts, and it's a vital dietary antioxidant.

Beta-carotene, also known as provitamin A, breaks down into highly active forms of vitamin A, which play an important role in vision, hearing, taste and smell. Best of all, studies have shown that when this hard-working carotene turns into one active vitamin A compound, it fights the free radical damage that causes cancer and heart disease.

In a Nurses Health Study of 87,000 women at Brigham and Women's Hospital in Boston, researchers found that nurses who ate 15 to 20 milligrams of beta-carotene (less than one cup of cooked carrots), along with another antioxidant, vitamin E, had 40 percent fewer heart attacks and strokes than women who consumed less than 6 milligrams a day. A Harvard study found similar benefits from beta-carotene. When 165 male physicians with signs of heart disease took beta-carotene supplements, they reduced by half their risk of strokes, heart attacks and death from heart disease, compared with a similar group of men who were not getting the supplements. To get these lifesaving results, the physicians took 50 milligrams of beta-carotene (the equivalent of about two cups of cooked carrots) every other day for six years.

For health-saving results, here's how to maximize beta-carotene—and its cousin carotenes—in your diet.

Eat the sunny colors. Orange-yellow produce will give you the most generous amounts of beta-carotene, ac-

PROTECTION FROM PARKINSON'S?

The trembling hands and wobbly gait caused by Parkinson's disease may result partly from free radical damage to nerve cells. And antioxidants may slow the disease's progression, early studies suggest. Most people who have Parkinson's show gradual symptoms of nerve damage, such as tremors, unusually slow movements and difficulty walking. But some doctors have found that medication can be postponed several years if newly diagnosed patients are given high doses of vitamins C and E.

While antioxidants do seem to protect nerve cells against free radical damage, however, there is no direct proof they can actually hold off Parkinson's, according to Tufts University researcher Dr. Mohsen Meydani. But a study has shown that one antioxidant may stave off symptoms that mimic Parkinson's. Dr. Meydani explains: "In people born unable to absorb fats, including fat-soluble E, the deficiency shows first in nerve-damage symptoms—trembling hands and trouble walking. Once these patients are injected with vitamin E, the symptoms disappear."

cording to Dr. Russell. While carrots are a great source of beta-carotene, it also comes in a lot of other colorful packages. "Don't forget dried apricots, sweet potatoes, red peppers and orange winter squash," he notes. Watermelon and cantaloupe are also good sources.

Gather the greens. The darker the better, when you want beta-carotene in your diet. Broccoli, spinach and kale are all good sources. And real greens-lovers also relish the taste of turnip greens, beet greens and collard greens, which top the list of dark-green sources.

Cook those veggies. You still get good nutrients and plenty of fiber from eating raw vegetables. But if you lightly steam the same vegetables, your body will get a lot more of their beta-carotene.

"Carotenes bind to other food components such as fiber, and when they're bound they're not as available to be absorbed," Dr. Russell says. "Cooking breaks that fiber/carotene bond."

Cooking carrots until they're just slightly tender, for instance, increases the availability of their carotene content three- or fourfold, according to Dr. Russell. And the availability of beta-carotene in broccoli doubles as soon as that vegetable is lightly cooked.

The key is to steam these vegetables in

a very small amount of water so they'll come out crunchy and not limp. (If you use enough water to cover the vegetables, you'll end up boiling them and pouring a considerable amount of their carotenes down the drain with the broth.)

For microwaving, use two tablespoons of water per cup of vegetables, and steam them in a covered dish. If you're cooking on a regular stove, use a steamer. Pour about an inch of water into the bottom of the pot, then steam the vegetables over medium heat.

Enjoy pumpkin year-round. "Pumpkin has an incredible amount of beta-carotene. It's really quite amazing," Dr. Russell notes.

A slice of pumpkin pie or pumpkin bread offers a hefty amount of beta-carotene, so enjoy it for a special dessert. You can count on finding canned pumpkin in stores year-round—with virtually the same amount of beta-carotene as fresh pumpkin.

Or prepare fresh pumpkin and store it, suggests Sooja Kim, R.D., Ph.D., scientific review administrator of the Nutrition Study Section at the National Institutes of Health (NIH). Cut open the pumpkin, scrape out the seeds and peel off the outer skin, then cut the pumpkin into chunks.

"Put it into a food processor and grind it," Dr. Kim advises. "It becomes a wonderful puree you can use fresh or frozen for pumpkin pies or soups."

Don't get hung up on iceberg. Iceberg lettuce is a loser when it comes to carotene counting, according to Dr. Russell. Expand your salad repertoire by choosing dark leafy greens such as spinach or Romaine lettuce, which have several times the beta-carotene content of iceberg. And anytime you add some raw broccoli or a few kale leaves, you're giving your salad a mighty beta boost.

If you have trouble getting used to the more vivid taste of these greens, blend them in with iceberg a bit at a time, gradually increasing the amount until they are your new salad staples.

Pump up your meat loaf. Tomato

sauce is a common ingredient in many homestyle meat loaf recipes—and there's nothing wrong with that. But as long as you're making your meat loaf healthier (less meat, more mixin's), why not pump up its antioxidant content?

"You can use pumpkin puree in meat loaf instead of tomato sauce," says Dr. Kim. The pumpkin is a new, unexpected taste—and surprisingly good with meat.

Dress your salad with betas. Pumpkin beats carrots and dark-green lettuce in the beta contest, but when you put them all together, they're an unbeatable combination. Once you have pumpkin puree in your freezer, you can easily make a quick, scrumptious pumpkin salad dressing in just a minute. "Mix pumpkin puree, oil, vinegar, garlic and your favorite herbs to taste," Dr. Kim recommends. Pour some on your favorite salad—and keep the rest in the fridge for next time.

Pick papayas. Tempt your palate with more exotic fruits like papayas, suggests Dr. Kim. These rich sources of beta-carotene are not always available in supermarkets, but when they are, you're in for a treat.

Papaya is a deep orange-colored tropical fruit with a very mild flavor that's a cross between honeydew melon and cantaloupe. To prepare it, just slice it open, remove the seeds and—for an extra zesty addition—sprinkle on some lime juice to complement its flavor.

"Sliced papaya is a good appetizer or dessert," Dr. Kim points out. The fruit doesn't become discolored when it's exposed to air, so you can prepare it way ahead of dinnertime, put it in a plastic bag and keep it in the refrigerator.

Mix it up with mangoes. Sweeter than papayas, high-beta mangoes are also becoming available in some supermarkets. Sliced, they're tasty on hot cereal.

"They're also a popular Thai dessert," Dr. Kim notes. "Just cut up a mango, *(continued on page 96)*

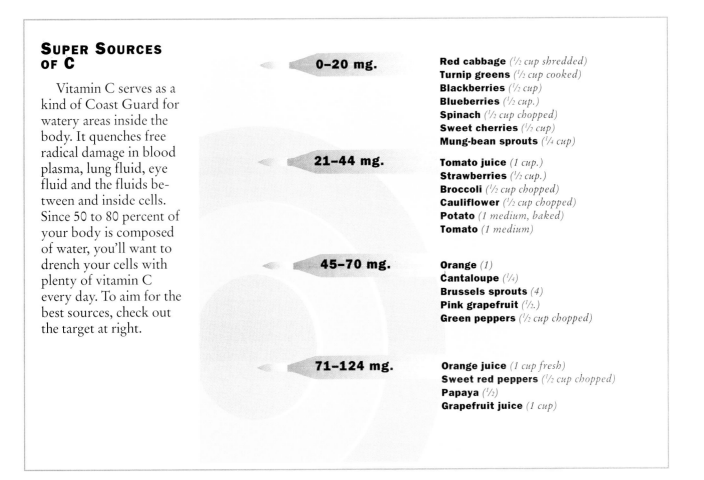

SUPER SOURCES OF C

Vitamin C serves as a kind of Coast Guard for watery areas inside the body. It quenches free radical damage in blood plasma, lung fluid, eye fluid and the fluids between and inside cells. Since 50 to 80 percent of your body is composed of water, you'll want to drench your cells with plenty of vitamin C every day. To aim for the best sources, check out the target at right.

0–20 mg.

Red cabbage (*½ cup shredded*)
Turnip greens (*½ cup cooked*)
Blackberries (*½ cup*)
Blueberries (*½ cup.*)
Spinach (*½ cup chopped*)
Sweet cherries (*½ cup*)
Mung-bean sprouts (*¼ cup*)

21–44 mg.

Tomato juice (*1 cup.*)
Strawberries (*½ cup.*)
Broccoli (*½ cup chopped*)
Cauliflower (*½ cup chopped*)
Potato (*1 medium, baked*)
Tomato (*1 medium*)

45–70 mg.

Orange (*1*)
Cantaloupe (*¼*)
Brussels sprouts (*4*)
Pink grapefruit (*½.*)
Green peppers (*½ cup chopped*)

71–124 mg.

Orange juice (*1 cup fresh*)
Sweet red peppers (*½ cup chopped*)
Papaya (*½*)
Grapefruit juice (*1 cup*)

Three Days to a Longer Life

How easy is it to pack age-erasing antioxidants into your daily diet? Very. To get started, try this three-day, high-antioxidant plan with menus for breakfast, lunch and dinner. All the meals include foods that are good sources of vitamin C, vitamin E and beta-carotene. This menu is just a starting point. As long as you get one serving of vegetables and one of fruit with every meal, you're on your way to fighting cancer and heart disease and boosting your immunity. For the vegetables and fruits in any of these meals, you can substitute your favorites, or browse the produce department for new varieties.

THE LONGEVITY MENU

	DAY 1	DAY 2	DAY 3
Breakfast	1 cup crisped rice cereal with 1 cup skim milk 1 mixed-grain English muffin with 1 tsp. margarine 1 pear	1 cup bran nuggets cereal with 3 Tbsp. raisins and 1 cup skim milk 2 slices enriched wheat toast with 2 tsp. margarine ½ papaya 1 cup skim milk	½ cup all-bran cereal with ½ cup sliced banana and 1 cup skim milk ½ cup fresh-squeezed orange juice 1 cinnamon roll with icing
Lunch	Sandwich made with 2 slices mixed-grain bread, 3 oz. smoked turkey breast, 2 leaves iceberg lettuce, 2 Tbsp. low-fat mayonnaise and ½ sliced tomato 2 kiwi fruits 6 oz. low-fat fruit yogurt 3 oz. broiled beef tenderloin	1 cup low-fat (1%) cottage cheese ½ pear ½ peach 2 whole-wheat rolls with 2 tsp. margarine and 2 Tbsp. jam or preserves	Sandwich made with 1 whole-wheat roll, 2 oz. smoked deli ham, 1 oz. low-fat Swiss cheese and 2 Tbsp. low-fat mayonnaise ½ cup canned plums in light syrup ½ mango ½ cup canned, sweetened grapefruit juice
Dinner	1 cup cooked long-grain brown rice Salad made with ½ cup Romaine lettuce, ½ tomato, 1 slice avocado and 2 Tbsp. Italian dressing 1 cup cooked broccoli 2 slices enriched whole-wheat bread with 2 tsp. margarine 1 cup skim milk *Antioxidant analysis: 333.9 mg. vitamin C; 32.8 IU vitamin E; 1.5 mg. beta-carotene*	3 ounces broiled haddock 1 cup mashed sweet potato Salad made with loose leaf lettuces, ¼ cup chopped raw mushrooms, ¼ cup diced tomato and 2 Tbsp. blue cheese dressing 1 cup skim milk *Antioxidant analysis: 244 mg. vitamin C; 29.9 IU vitamin E; 23.5 mg. beta-carotene*	3 oz. baked salmon 2 whole-wheat rolls with 2 Tbsp. margarine ½ cup baby lima beans Salad with ¼ head iceberg lettuce, ¼ cup raw carrots, ¼ cup chopped spinach and 2 Tbsp. Russian dressing 1 cup skim milk ½ cup cooked dried apricots *Antioxidant analysis: 207.3 mg. vitamin C; 35.8 IU vitamin E; 9.2 mg. beta-carotene*

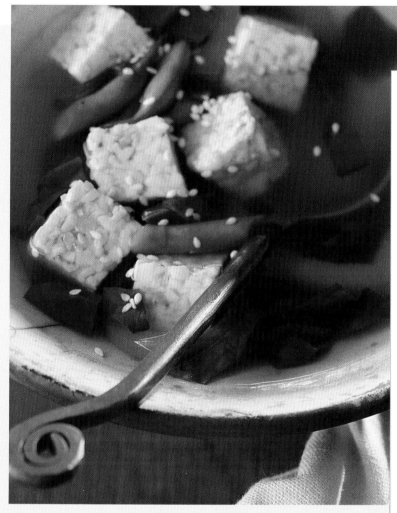

Make the most of miso, which has been linked to a reduced risk of stomach cancer, when you make a miso bean soup that includes high-C vegetables.

YOUTH-STYLE SOUP

With a tasty base of low-sodium vegetable stock, this oriental-style soup is a veritable foundation of youth. The spinach and sweet red peppers contribute a good supply of the antioxidants beta-carotene and vitamin C. The miso paste used in this fragrant soup can be found in most Asian markets and health food stores.

This recipe also calls for tempeh, which is a high-protein "cake" made from soybeans. Look for it in the freezer section of health food stores. (You may also substitute tofu.)

Miso Bean Soup

3 cups low-sodium vegetable stock
3 cups water
1 cup cubed tempeh
1 tablespoon miso
1 cup cut (1" pieces) green beans
1 cup coarsely chopped spinach
1 cup thinly sliced sweet red peppers
1 teaspoon minced fresh ginger
1 tablespoon toasted sesame seeds

In a 3-quart saucepan over medium-high heat, bring the stock and water to a boil. Add the tempeh and cook for 2 minutes.

Ladle out about ¼ cup of the liquid and place it in a cup. Add the miso and mix well to dissolve it. Set aside.

Reduce the heat to medium. Stir in the beans, spinach, peppers and ginger. Cook for 5 minutes, or just until the vegetables are tender.

Immediately before serving, add the miso mixture. Simmer for 2 minutes, but don't allow the soup to boil. Serve sprinkled with the sesame seeds.

Makes 4 servings.

Per serving: 148 calories, 5.8 g. fat (33% of calories), 1.8 g. dietary fiber, 0 mg. cholesterol, 322 mg. sodium.

KEEP YOUR SIGHTS ON C LOSS

While many raw vegetables are chock-full of vitamin C, some of that youth-preserving vitamin gets lost during cooking.

How much depends on how you cook those veggies. When nutritionists measured the vitamin C loss in broccoli, for instance, they found that the amount that's lost during preparation can differ drastically, depending on the cooking method used. Here's how the different cooking methods measure up.

Cooking Method	Vitamin C (mg./1 spear)	Vitamin C Lost in Cooking
Before cooking	141	—
Microwaving	120	15%
Pressure cooking	113	20%
Steaming	99	30%
Boiling	63	55%

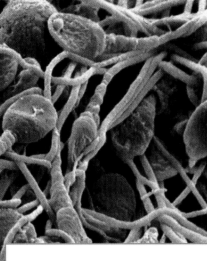

Vitamin C helps protect sperm, making it stronger and more plentiful.

AN ORANGE A DAY IS GOOD FOR DAD

There's good news for nutrition-conscious fathers-to-be: Keeping an eye on your vitamin C intake can be a lifesaver for the l'il nipper who's going to occupy the highchair.

Researchers have found that fathers' high-C diets can make the difference between healthy offspring and babies who have an increased risk of birth defects and hereditary diseases.

The amount of vitamin C in just one orange a day may protect sperm's genetic material from the kind of damage that leads to these congenital problems, say researchers at the University of California at Berkeley. Damage to sperm increased 91 percent in men on a low-vitamin-C diet that supplied just 5 milligrams a day, the researchers report. But once higher levels of vitamin C (60 or 250 milligrams) were restored to their diets, the damage declined.

What's the link? Vitamin C is naturally found in high concentrations in sperm and is generally believed to protect the genetic material in sperm from free radical attacks.

For smokers, even larger doses of vitamin C are needed to defend against the destructive punch of nicotine. Because nicotine helps destroy vitamin C, smokers need additional C to offset the loss. To find out the effects of vitamin C on nicotine-damaged sperm cells, male fertility expert Earl Dawson, Ph.D., of the University of Texas Medical School at Galveston, did a study with 75 young male smokers. Two-thirds received either 200 or 1,000 milligrams of vitamin C every day for a month, and the remaining third got a placebo (a blank pill).

All the men, the tests showed, had sperm that was damaged by nicotine. But the men who got the most vitamin C had the least damage. The high-C subjects also produced more sperm, according to Dr. Dawson, and their sperm were better swimmers.

then mix it with cooked rice, a little brown sugar and lime juice."

For an incredible treat anytime, Dr. Kim recommends a mango "smoothie." Slice up some mangoes, put the pieces in a blender with a cup of skim milk and a ripe banana and blend until smooth.

Pick the peculiar. If your supermarket has seasonal fruits you haven't seen before, remember that every new color means a new source of beta-carotene. In fall, for instance, you'll find red-skinned mellow-sweet pomegranates in many supermarkets and Asian grocery stores. Just peel and eat the seeds. Their little burst of juice contains vitamins C and E along with beta-carotene.

Also in fall, keep your eyes open for acorn-shaped persimmons, which can be mashed and frozen for later. Try both the soft Hachiya and firm Fuyu varieties. Dr. Kim recommends that you use the persimmon mash to replace fattening oils in cake and muffin recipes. Persimmons are also good for desserts, fruit cocktail and salad.

THE VITAL VITAMIN

Vitamin C is a vital ingredient in the formation of collagen, the biological "glue" that binds your cells together. Without healthy collagen, skin heals poorly and sensitive tissues, such as the gums, can bleed easily. Vitamin C also helps your body absorb other vital nutrients, such as iron and calcium.

And now there's compelling evidence that vitamin C may be a wellspring of the fountain of youth. Vitamin C is actually your body's first line of defense against early aging. When oxidants are added to human blood, vitamin C is the first antioxidant to cancel them out, before any of the other antioxidants go to work.

In a study at the University of California at Berkeley, researchers removed vitamin C from the blood plasma of healthy volunteers and then added the kinds of oxidants that cause cell breakdown. After the vitamin C was removed, they found, oxidation picked up rapidly. But when they put the vitamin C back in, the plasma was again protected from oxidation.

Because vitamin C is water soluble, it's generally not stored in the body for long. Excess vitamin C is regularly passed in the urine rather than stored away, according to the NIA's Dr. Starke-Reed.

"Vitamin C is something you have to consume every day, by eating citrus fruits and other high-C foods. And the older you get, the more important this is," says Dr. Starke-Reed.

From recent studies, it looks as if a modest amount of vitamin C can make a difference in life expectancy. In fact, as little as 300 milligrams a day seems to tilt the scales in our favor. To get that much, you'd need to drink a cup of orange juice and eat one cup of cantaloupe chunks and a one-cup serving of steamed broccoli sometime during the day.

Here are some other ways to keep your cells chock-full of vitamin C.

Stock your OJ by the week. After one week, orange juice that's been opened and stored in its own carton or a plastic pitcher in the fridge loses just 12 percent of its vitamin C, say researchers from the U.S. Citrus and Subtropical Products Laboratory in Winter Haven, Florida. But after two weeks, the loss jumps to around 35 percent. If you drink one small cup of orange juice daily, buy just a quart. Better yet, squeeze your own when you need it! And if you mix your juice from frozen concentrate, fix small batches regularly for maximum C. When used promptly, other fresh or frozen juices contain similar levels of vitamin C (about 120 milligrams per cup), so just enjoy your favorite.

Throw citrus in your salads. Who says everything in a salad has to be a vegetable? Add orange and grapefruit sections to your green salads, not only for an extra burst of C but also for more of the valuable fiber whole fruits offer. Or vary your salad routine with all-fruit salads, using plenty of cantaloupe and honeydew melon, strawberries and kiwi fruit in addition to citrus.

Prep some peppers. While you're cutting carrot sticks for lunch, also remember to slice up some sweet peppers for a big vitamin C punch. Both red and green peppers are a good source of vitamin C, but the reds take the prize, packing more than double the antioxidant of the green variety. Slice a pepper lengthwise in hefty bite-size chunks and include them in your snack pack for home, car or office. Of course, they're also great in salads. And those long, curved slices make good dipping sticks for your favorite low-fat dip.

Don't let your C go up in smoke. As long as you're eating more vitamin C–rich foods, you can do yourself a favor by avoiding smoke-filled restaurants. It's long been known that people who smoke reduce their own vitamin C levels. The new wrinkle is that people who light up might be zapping your stores of the vitamin, too.

Researchers measured levels of vitamin C in the plasma of smokers, passive smokers (nonsmokers who breathed smoky air about 20 hours a week) and nonsmokers who kept their air mostly

FOODS TO EXPAND YOUR LIFE SPAN

Strawberries, grapefruit and broccoli not only delight your palate, they may also "C" you into a longer life.

Why? These fruits and vegetables are especially rich in super-antioxidant vitamin C. And a large study from the University of California School of Public Health has shown that consuming more vitamin C may reward you with more years of life.

A total of 11,348 adults participated in the national nutrition survey. Three groups of men and women were tracked for an average of 15 years. Group I took in less than 50 milligrams of vitamin C each day from food, Group II took in about 150 milligrams daily (also from food), and Group III got a total of over 300 milligrams from both food and supplement sources.

Over the 15-year span of the study, researchers found that the high-C men in Group III had a much lower death rate than the low-C men from Group I. In fact, judging from this study, men who get plenty of vitamin C in their diet can expect to live 6 years longer than those who consume very little.

Women also benefit from C, though less dramatically, according to the study. The life span of the women in Group III—the ones who got over 300 milligrams a day from food and supplements—was an average of two years longer than that of the women in Group I.

Whether you're scaling the heights or turning over the garden, vitamin E may be able to help you reduce that day-after muscle soreness.

clear. It turns out that where there was smoke (even someone else's), there were diminished levels of vitamin C—even though all three groups got roughly the same amount of it from their diets. So if you want the full benefits of the vitamin C in your diet, you'll want to avoid smoke-filled places as well as smoking.

VITAMIN E TO THE RESCUE

It doesn't take much vitamin E to make a difference. In your body this antioxidant may be the most powerful nutrient there is for preventing chronic illness and premature aging, researchers say. Vitamin E is so promising that numerous studies are under way to determine exactly what it does and how it works. Already, the news is good.

Vitamin E behaves like the Wild West sheriff of your body, shooting it out with free radicals before they stake their claim to your cells. When you are exposed to a variety of environmental carcinogens, ranging from tobacco smoke and pesticides to ozone and radiation, the oxidation process picks up its pace and increases your risk of cancer. But several studies now suggest that vitamin E meets these toxic compounds at the boundaries of your cells and may prevent them from causing cancerous tumors.

Take ozone, for example, which is a key component of smog. In a laboratory experiment, researchers at the New England Medical Center in Boston exposed cells pretreated with vitamin E to ozone and demonstrated that vitamin E made the cells resistant to free radical attack.

That's how vitamin E seems to protect cells most, other studies indicate. It helps keep cell walls intact so toxins can't enter, and it makes it hard for free radicals to swoop in.

Vitamin E also boosts your immune power—and that's a vital part of your body's defenses against cancer. One study directed by Dr. Meydani at the Human Nutrition Research Center at Tufts showed that vitamin E supplements clearly improved the immune response in healthy adults. This finding is believed to be particularly important because our immune system usually weakens as we age.

Because vitamin E has an antioxidant action, researchers also think it could help ease youth-sapping rheumatoid arthritis—and some animal studies seem to confirm this. When people have this kind of arthritis, it's because free radical molecules have rushed to the aching joint, attracted by the presence of bacteria. And those free radicals produce painful inflammation. But if you get plenty of vitamin E, researchers surmise, you may be able to reduce the effects of arthritis as you age.

Researchers are also trying to find out whether vitamin E can help prevent or alleviate certain kinds of cancers and some common problems of aging such as Parkinson's disease and cataracts.

WRINKLES CAN WAIT

Ninety percent of wrinkles are caused by the sun's radiation. In addition to using sunscreen faithfully, you can get extra wrinkle protection with daily doses of vitamin E (400 international units) and the trace mineral selenium (100 micrograms), research suggests.

While some researchers say supplements help, others claim that only vitamin E applied to the skin will do any good. It is found in many skin lotions and sunscreens—just read the ingredients list on the labels.

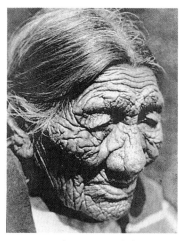

Mapping the power of the sun's rays, the face of this 62-year-old Native American woman reveals what sunlight does to skin.

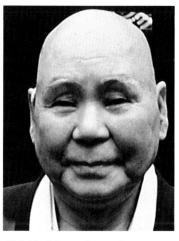

Shielded from the sun's rays, a 91-year-old Tibetan monk has the unwrinkled face of a much younger man.

GETTING E'S WITH EASE

Food sources might give you all the vitamin E you need to maintain health, but they're not a sure thing. The Daily Value (DV) is 30 international units—and some diets do provide that much.

There's a problem with food sources, however. Vitamin E tends to hang out in some unsavory places—chiefly in foods that contain polyunsaturated fats. Nuts, dairy products, eggs and certain vegetable oils are prime examples of high-fat foods that happen to contain an abundance of vitamin E. And eating too much of these fatty foods promotes obesity, warns Dr. Meydani, who does vitamin E research at Tufts.

Instead, he suggests, to get the full rejuvenating benefits of this powerhouse nutrient, ask your doctor about vitamin E supplements. For most people, a daily dose of 100 to 400 international units would help promote health and longevity, according to Dr. Meydani.

But even if you do take supplements, there are other ways to get vitamin E in your diet without overdoing your daily fat intake. Here are some tactics that get the nod from nutritionists.

Sow seeds in your salads. Sunflower seeds are generous providers of vitamin E. Sprinkle them in your salads for a burst of nutty flavor and use them as nutritious snacks, says NIH dietitian Dr. Kim. There's one drawback, however: You may take in too much fat if you eat more than a small handful.

Scoop up some youth. Around Halloween, we scoop out and throw away enough pumpkin seeds to make most of America a younger nation. Those flat, slippery seeds surrounded by stringy pumpkin innards are chock-full of vitamin E. And they're easy to prepare for snacks.

Wash the seeds in a strainer and dry them on a towel. Then scatter them around a baking sheet and roast them slowly at 150°F until they're crunchy. They're filling snacks, with just a slight snap of pumpkin flavor in every fibrous, vitamin E–filled bite.

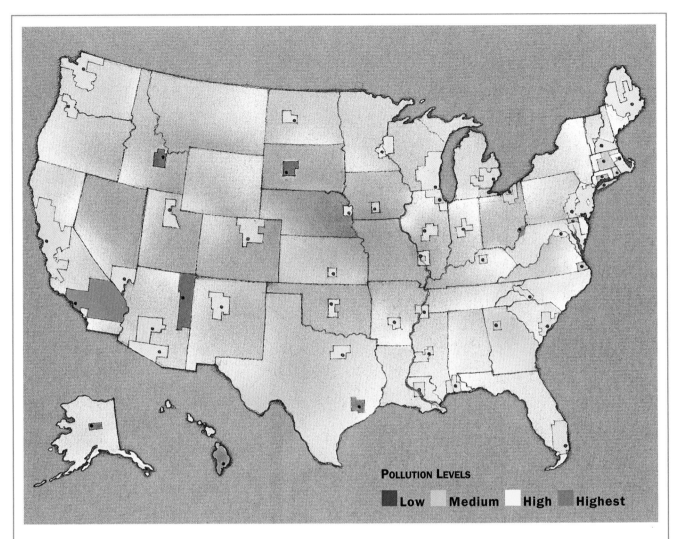

POLLUTION LEVELS

■ Low ■ Medium ■ High ■ Highest

PROTECT YOUR LUNGS WITH VITAMIN E

Does your hometown rank among America's most polluted cities? This map compares the levels of pollution—as measured by ozone concentrations—in some cities throughout the United States.

Vitamin E helps your lungs fend off damage from the toxins found in most air pollution, numerous studies have shown. So if you are in a high-pollution area, be sure to keep track of the vitamin E you're getting. Your cells need that extra protection.

Galena, Alaska	Honolulu, Hawaii,	Howe, Idaho	Indian Wells, Arizona
Kadoka, South Dakota			

Albuquerque, New Mexico	Denver, Colorado	Memphis, Tennessee	Portland, Oregon
Alexandria, Virginia	Des Moines, Iowa	Miami, Florida	Providence, Rhode Island
Bangor, Maine	Detroit, Michigan	Milwaukee, Wisconsin	Salt Lake City, Utah
Bismarck, North Dakota	Indianapolis, Indiana	Minneapolis, Minnesota	San Francisco, California
Boston, Massachusetts	Jackson, Mississippi	Mobile, Alabama	Seattle, Washington
Charleston, South Carolina	Las Vegas, Nevada	Oklahoma City, Oklahoma	Springfield, Illinois
Charlotte, North Carolina	Lexington, Kentucky	Omaha, Nebraska	Tucson, Arizona
Concord, New Hampshire	Little Rock, Arkansas	Philadelphia, Pennsylvania	Wichita, Kansas

Atlanta, Georgia	Chicago, Illinois	New Haven, Connecticut	Phoenix, Arizona
Baltimore, Maryland	Cleveland, Ohio	New York, New York	St. Louis, Missouri
Baton Rouge, Louisiana	Dallas, Texas	Norfolk, Virginia	Worcester, Massachusetts

Athens, Ohio	Houston, Texas	Los Angeles, California	

Peanuts and almonds are good sources of vitamin E, too, but as with sunflower seeds, you should go easy because of the fat. "As always, moderation is the best policy," cautions Dr. Kim.

Eat your weeds. For fans of "found food," there could be a good vitamin E source right around your yard. The common plant purslane—usually considered a weed by American gardeners—is a potent antioxidant. It contains six times the vitamin E of spinach (and for heart health, hefty amounts of omega-3 fatty acids). Try steaming the leaves lightly, just as you'd cook spinach. Fresh purslane can also be tossed in salads.

Sow the germ of youth. Wheat germ is the vitamin- and mineral-rich embryo of the wheat berry that is removed when flour is refined from whole wheat to white. It's a good source of vitamin E, with four milligrams per $\frac{1}{4}$ cup. Try it toasted or raw on frozen yogurt. Wheat germ also makes a healthy addition to casseroles, meat loaf, bread, muffins and pancakes.

YOUNG-FOR-LIFE BODY BUILDERS

A young body deserves a sturdy frame—and that means getting plenty of calcium in your diet. But along with calcium, you need plenty of vitamin D. Without it your bones won't harden, no matter how much calcium you offer them. And although neither calcium nor vitamin D is an antioxidant, they are still top "youth nutrients."

You can get plenty of vitamin D in your diet from a variety of low-fat products. Nonfat milk, along with many breads and cereals, is usually fortified with D. Just two cups of fortified skim milk, for example, supplies 50 percent of the DV for vitamin D.

Another simple source of vitamin D is sunlight—your skin manufactures it when exposed to the sun's ultraviolet light. But getting adequate amounts of vitamin D can be a problem for faithful users of sunscreen.

Experts agree it's very important for children and young adults to apply sunscreen before going outdoors for long periods. They're outside every day, so it's unlikely that sunscreen use will lead to vitamin D deficiency.

The situation is a bit different for people who are older. The elderly don't make as much vitamin D in their skin, and if they always use a sunscreen, they may not have enough for good bone health. In most cases, though, five to ten minutes a week of sun exposure without sunscreen will provide the benefits with little risk of damage.

As for the core ingredient of bone-building, all-important calcium, experts recommend that most people get at least 1,000 milligrams a day. (Exceptions: Men and women under the age of 25 should get 1,200 milligrams per day, and the National Osteoporosis Foundation recommends that postmenopausal women aim for 1,500 milligrams daily if they're not on estrogen replacement therapy.)

The best sources of calcium by far are nonfat or low-fat dairy products (for more detail about these sources, see chapter 11). And several are fortified with vitamin D, making it easy to get both vital bone builders at once. Eight ounces of nonfat yogurt, for instance, offer 452 milligrams of calcium, while a cup of skim milk has 302 milligrams.

Sardines also offer rich amounts of calcium, because you also eat the tiny calcium-rich bones in the sardines. Just seven sardines provide 321 milligrams of calcium. Similarly, three ounces of pink salmon, with bones, supply 181 milligrams.

Once you turn to plant sources, the calcium numbers start to slide—but vegetables still offer good amounts. Half-cup servings of Chinese cabbage (bok choy), mustard greens, kale and pinto beans have amounts ranging from 41 to 86 milligrams. Spinach also contains plenty of calcium (122 milligrams per $\frac{1}{2}$ cup), but it's not recommended as a good source: The oxalic acid it also contains makes the calcium unavailable to your body.

Two Big Reasons for B's

For the crowd that wants to stay young, the B vitamins provide a wide range of benefits. Research has shown that foods high in B vitamins can help reduce the risk of premature heart disease. And it's long been known that people need B vitamins to help keep their memories sharp and to solve abstract problems.

B's FOR THE YOUNG AT HEART

Homocysteine is a substance you've probably never heard of. But rest assured you'll be hearing plenty in the next few years. The fact is, in people with very elevated blood levels of homocysteine (a condition called *hyperhomocysteinemia*), the risk of premature vascular disease is 30 times greater than for those with normal levels. And even in people who don't have this condition, higher levels of homocysteine have been linked to greater heart disease risk.

In the Physicians' Health Study (the study that yielded the news that aspirin prevents heart attacks), researchers found that people with the highest levels of homocysteine had a three times higher risk of heart attack.

"Obviously, for people with a high level of homocysteine, it's important to bring that level down," says Meir Stampfer, M.D., professor of epidemiology and nutrition at the Harvard School of Public Health, who led the study. "But even at average levels, it may turn out to be a worthwhile idea to lower levels further."

Here's where the B vitamins come into play: Folic acid, B_6 and B_{12} all play a role in converting homocysteine into nontoxic compounds. When your body is deficient in one of these three B's, it cannot efficiently alter homocysteine.

Researchers agree that B vitamins are no magic bullet against homocysteine, or for that matter, heart disease. "For one thing, B vitamins will ordinarily do nothing to correct a genetic enzyme deficiency," says Rowena Matthews, Ph.D., professor of biological chemistry at the University of Michigan Biophysics Research Division.

Then there's the matter of whether the three B's—which researchers strongly suspect can lower homocysteine—will actually prove, in turn, to lower heart attack risk. "We expect they will," says Jacob Selhub, Ph.D., of the USDA Human Nutrition Research Center on Aging at Tufts University. "But we don't know that. Clinical trials must be conducted."

Researchers agree, though, that until more is known about the relationship among homocysteine, B vitamins and heart disease, your best bet seems to be to make sure you're getting enough B's.

Folic acid (also known as folate) can be found in orange juice, greens like broccoli and spinach, and legumes, including navy beans, lima beans and kidney beans. Rich sources of B_6 include bananas, baked potatoes (with the skin), peas and avocados. Besides these natural sources, many cereals are fortified with 25 percent of the Daily Value (DV) for both folic acid and vitamin B_6 per serving. (Check the labels to find ones that are high in these vitamins.)

Vitamin B_{12}, however, poses a nutritional dilemma. Some of the best sources (beef liver and lamb kidney, for example) are also high in saturated fat and cholesterol. But that doesn't mean you can't get plenty of this vitamin with some careful menu planning. For example, a three-ounce slice of lean beef, a bowl of B_{12}-fortified cereal and an eight-ounce glass of skim milk will provide nearly all the DV for B_{12}. Fermented soy products are also rich in B_{12}.

For those who are concerned that they may not be getting enough B vitamins in their diets, Dr. Stampfer recommends a multivitamin supplement that provides the recommended levels of B_6,

B_{12}, folic acid and other vital nutrients.

The DV for vitamin B_6 is 2 milligrams; for B_{12}, it's 6 micrograms and for folic acid, 0.4 milligram. Supplements of these B vitamins should not greatly exceed these recommendations due to the risk of side effects.

The findings on homocysteine and heart disease may go a long way toward explaining heart disease that occurs when none of the standard risk factors—smoking, high blood pressure or elevated cholesterol—are present.

B's for Brain Food

Numerous studies suggest that very mild vitamin deficiencies play a part in many of the frustrations older people face, such as forgetfulness and even more serious problems that can look like senility. And the B vitamins may be key factors.

Harvard and Tufts University researchers have found that low (even slightly low) levels of B_{12} and folate are associated with depression in the elderly. Researchers believe one reason older folks are prone to having low levels of these nutrients is that they make less stomach acid than younger people do. Without enough acid, even if you're eating a balanced diet, your body can't absorb the depression-fighting nutrients efficiently.

Other studies showed that healthy older people with low levels of folate, B_{12} and riboflavin (vitamin B_2) in their blood scored poorly on tests of memory and abstract thinking. People with Alzheimer's disease are especially likely to be low in B_{12}, say researchers from the University of Toronto.

And a low-B diet won't just make you foggy and forgetful; it can make you downright cranky. Too little folate (found in wheat germ, beans and other legumes) has been linked to irritability and even paranoia, doctors say.

It's not hard to bolster your brain-power with more B vitamins, however. Fortified cereals, chicken and fish boast generous amounts of B_6 and B_{12}.

When you serve up your brain food buffet, don't forget iron and zinc. One preliminary study of 34 iron-deficient women showed that those who took iron and zinc supplements improved notably on tests of short-term visual memory. Iron was also found to improve verbal memory by 20 percent.

Lean meats can beef up your zinc and iron levels. Researchers say, however, that there is no evidence of any benefit from taking extra iron and zinc, and too much may be harmful.

A Banquet of B Vitamins

Your memory, mood and math skills all depend on B vitamins. You'll need enough of these brain-boosting nutrients to ensure peak mental powers as you age, researchers say.

Food	Portion	Vitamin Amount
Vitamin B$_{12}$		
Clams	20 small (about 3 oz.)	89 mcg.
Atlantic mackerel, baked or broiled	3 oz.	16 mcg.
Atlantic herring, baked or broiled	3 oz.	11.2 mcg.
Tuna, baked or broiled	3 oz.	9.3 mcg.
Blue crab, steamed	3 oz.	6.2 mcg.
Sockeye salmon, canned, drained	3 oz.	0.3 mcg.
Vitamin B$_6$		
Banana	1 (about 4 oz.)	0.7 mg.
Potato, baked	1 (about 7 oz.)	0.7 mg.
Chick-peas, canned	1/2 cup	0.6 mg.
Prune juice, canned	1 cup	0.6 mg.
Turkey, white meat, roasted	3 oz.	0.5 mg.
Carrot juice, canned	3/4 cup	0.4 mg.
Folate		
Lentils, boiled	1/2 cup	179 mcg.
Pinto beans, boiled	1/2 cup	146 mcg.
Baby lima beans, boiled	1/2 cup	136 mcg.
Black beans, boiled	1/2 cup	128 mcg.
Kidney beans, boiled	1/2 cup	114 mcg.
Wheat germ, toasted	1/4 cup	100 mcg.
Riboflavin		
Chicken liver, simmered	3 oz.	1.5 mg.
Nonfat yogurt	1 cup	0.5 mg.
Skim milk	1 cup	0.3 mg.
Cocoa	1 cup	0.4 mg.
Low-fat (1%) milk	1 cup	0.4 mg.
Swiss cheese	1 oz.	0.1 mg.

Dietary Breakthroughs for Cancer Prevention

Inside your body are some 50 trillion cells, the building blocks of your bones, brain, nerves and everything else that makes you you. As time goes by, every one of these cells will grow, mature and then divide, forming two new cells to take its place.

In an average adult, nearly one trillion blood cells die every day and must be replaced. Most of the time, that's exactly what happens: The birth of new cells precisely matches the death of old ones.

Should a cell become damaged, however—as a result of things such as radiation, pollution, cigarette smoke or even bad luck—the balance can suddenly and dangerously go awry. "Tumor cells don't recognize or accept the signal to stop multiplying," says Carl M. Mansfield, M.D., professor and chairman of the Department of Radiation, Oncology and Nuclear Medicine at Thomas Jefferson University Hospital in Philadelphia.

A cell that normally divides once a week, for example, could conceivably double, triple or even quadruple its numbers in a matter of days. Each one of the new cells is also abnormal—and just as prolific. Over time, one damaged cell can become thousands, then millions and then billions. The result, says Dr. Mansfield, is cancer—cell growth and multiplication that's out of control.

Although experts have identified many factors that can lead to cancer, there's one that really stands out—and it's in your hands.

THE FOOD FACTOR

Recently there's been increasing evidence that diet—either eating too many bad foods or not getting enough good ones—can be a key player in this mortal game.

"Dietary factors probably account for up to 35 percent of all cancers," reports Edward Trapido, Sc.D., chief of epidemiology at the University of Miami School of Medicine.

In one large study, scientists analyzed the data from a dozen smaller studies that involved 10,000 women worldwide. The relationship was consistent: As saturated fat intake went up, so did the risk for breast cancer. The reverse occurred with fruits and vegetables: The more vitamin C from these foods the women got in their diets, the lower their cancer risk.

Protection that works for the goose is also good for the gander. Italian and Swiss researchers found that men who ate seven servings of vegetables a week were less likely to get prostate cancer than men who ate six or less.

SMALL CHANGES, DRAMATIC BENEFITS

In light of these and many other studies, the U.S. Department of Agriculture, the surgeon general and the National Cancer Institute (NCI) have called on Americans to reduce their intake of dietary fat to no more than 30

CELLULAR WAR

Cancer is a daunting opponent, but a well-nourished immune system can fight back with killer T-cells. Experts aren't sure how the process works, but an encounter between a cancer cell and a killer T-cell may result in the cancer cell's death—before it grows into a tumor.

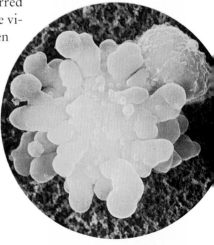

Vastly outweighed in battle, a killer T-cell attacks a large tumor cell, which attempts to defend itself by forming blisters on its surface.

percent of total calories (many health-care experts recommend an even lower target of 25 percent) and to eat at least five servings of fruits and vegetables every day.

Unfortunately, we're not even close. In one survey of over 11,000 adults, an estimated 45 percent reported having no fruit or juice on a certain day, while 22 percent said they had no vegetables. Only 9 percent had the five servings of fruits and vegetables recommended by the NCI and other medical experts.

"The word is getting out, but we need to show people that it's not so hard to do," says Bruce J. Trock, Ph.D., epidemiologist at the Lombardi Cancer Center at Georgetown University Medical Center in Washington, D.C. "It doesn't mean you have to give up meat or eggs or cheese or any of that stuff. You just need to eat a little less of them, and to increase your intake of some of these other things."

SLIM PROTECTION

Researchers have long suspected that cancer and fat—whether the fat is on your plate or your waist—are not a healthy pair. In a study at the University of Buffalo, for example, researchers found that people who got more than 33 percent of their daily calories from fat had 2½ times the risk of developing cancer of the larynx, compared with those whose fat intake was about 21 percent. Being overweight may also boost the risk for cancers of the colon, breast, prostate, gallbladder, uterus and ovaries.

Experts agree that the upper limit of fat intake should be between 25 and 30 percent of calories—the same limit that will help you lose weight and improve your arterial health. But most Americans get over 35 percent of their calories from fat. "It's difficult to study the effects of dietary fat in the Western population because we're all eating so much fat," comments NCI epidemiologist Nancy Potischman, Ph.D. This is why researchers often look outside our borders, to compare U.S. cancer rates with

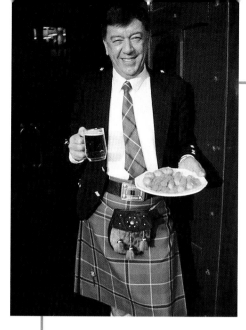

A Scot savors a traditional pub meal—typically high in fat, low in fiber and devoid of green vegetables. It's a diet that raises cancer risk, studies show.

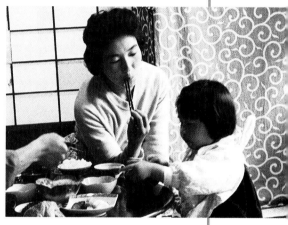

Many Japanese enjoy diets based on rice, vegetables and fish, with scant amounts of meat and fats. The result is one of the lowest cancer rates in the world.

THE CULTURE OF CANCER

For a revealing glimpse of the cancer/nutrition connection, consider two countries: Scotland and Japan. In Scotland, fat consumption is high, and nearly 20 percent of men and 13 percent of women say they almost never eat green vegetables. About 4 out of every 1,000 people die of cancer. In Japan, where rice and vegetables are served with almost every meal, the number of deaths from cancer is closer to 3 out of every 1,000.

those in countries where people eat little fat. Comparisons show that diet makes a significant difference in cancer rates.

In Japan, for example, where the typical diet is long on rice and vegetables and short on fats, annual death rates from cancer are much lower than they are in the United States. In fact, the death rate from cancer in the United States is about 16 percent higher than it is in Japan.

(continued on page 108)

Reducing Breast Cancer Risk

It's hard to accept the idea that your own body produces a substance that can encourage a group of tiny breast cells to form cancerous clusters. But researchers believe that's exactly what happens. "There's overwhelming evidence that the female hormone estrogen plays a central role in causing breast cancer," says Ronald Ross, M.D., professor of preventive medicine at the University of Southern California School of Medicine in Los Angeles.

Evidence suggests that the less a woman is exposed to her own reproductive hormones, the lower her risk for developing breast cancer. That's why experts are now recommending that all women maintain their ideal body weight and eat a well-balanced, low-fat diet with plenty of fruits, vegetables and whole grains. This—along with things such as breast-feeding and regular exercise—can substantially lower the amount of estrogen in your body, and with it the risk for developing cancer.

In one study, for example, 62 women were placed on diets containing ½ to 1 ounce of fiber—in the form of wheat, oats or corn—a day. After two months on the wheat-fiber diet, there was a significant drop in estrone, a type of estrogen implicated in raising cancer risk. (Oat and corn fiber had little effect.)

"This fits well with what we've seen in foreign countries, where fat intakes are similar to ours but rates of cancer are much lower," says David P. Rose, M.D., D.Sc., chief of the Division of Nutrition and Endocrinology of the Naylor Dana Institute of the American Health Foundation in Valhalla, New York, who was a coauthor of the study. "It's probably related to their high fiber intake."

CANCER "PHYTERS"

Can you eat your way to good health? Researchers say yes, particularly if you reach deep into nature's medicine chest—the produce section at your supermarket.

Studies show that a number of fruits and vegetables contain phytochemicals. These naturally occurring compounds include sulforaphane (found in vegetables such as broccoli), phytosterols (found in soybeans) and isoflavones (found in beans) that may help block tumors before they get started.

In laboratory studies at Johns Hopkins University in Baltimore, rats treated with a high dose of the synthetic form of sulforaphane were only about one-quarter as likely to develop breast tumors as those that were not treated. Researchers also found that sulforaphane delayed the onset of cancer and kept the size and number of any tumors comparatively small. They speculate that sulforaphane may increase the body's output of enzymes that help protect the cells against cancer-causing compounds.

When you eat fruits and vegetables, of course, you're getting a lot more than just a single active ingredient. You're also getting fiber and a host of important vitamins and minerals. Studies show that those who get the least fruits, juices and vegetables are the ones most at risk for many cancers, including breast cancer.

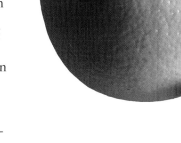

But while a high-fiber diet is part of the solution, it's not the only solution. Just as important for a woman's health is cutting back on the fat, says Sherwood L. Gorbach, M.D., professor of community health and medicine at Tufts University School of Medicine in Boston. In order to lower the risk of breast cancer, the maximum fat in the diet should be about 20 or 25 percent of total calories, experts say. "In countries where women eat a low-fat, high-fiber diet, they have lower estrogen levels and lower breast cancer risk," says Dr. Gorbach.

And don't forget the fruits and vegetables. Researchers find that those who generally eat at least five servings of fruits and vegetables a day reduce their risk of breast cancer.

Estradiol

Protein globulin

Broccoli. Like brussels sprouts, cabbage and kale, this vegetable contains a variety of cancer-fighting compounds that help estrogen change into harmless estrogen derivatives that are excreted from the body.

In a balanced system: The form of estrogen called estradiol is trapped by protein globulins. (Normally, there are plenty of globulin molecules to trap the unneeded molecules of estradiol.) The result: Relatively little estradiol in breast tissues and a low risk for cancer.

Garlic. This pungent bulb contains sulfur compounds that reduce the body's output of estradiol, which is the most potent form of estrogen. The sulfur compounds also "neutralize" excess estradiol that's already in the bloodstream and help slow tumor growth by enhancing the body's natural defenses.

Cancer development: Should there be an increase in estradiol or a decline in the amount of globulin available to mop it up, the risk for breast cancer rises. Fat tissue is a good source of estrogen— and since the American diet is so rich in fat and calories, this imbalance of estradiol and globulin is common.

Orange and lemon peel. Both contain limonene, a compound that boosts the efficiency of the body's protein globulins, which help eliminate surplus estradiol from the body. Limonene also activates enzymes that can destroy cancer cell membranes.

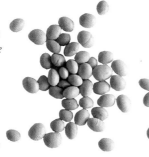

Estradiol at tumor site

Tumor growth: Once estradiol molecules latch on to specific sites—called receptors—on breast cells, they begin sending signals to the genetic material inside. This can cause the cells to begin dividing at an accelerated rate, possibly causing cancer.

Soybeans. These contain a number of phytochemicals, including genistein. Genistein has effects similar to tamoxifen, a drug used to prevent breast cancer.

"Their rates of things like breast and colon cancer were among the lowest in the world," says Dr. Trock. He adds, however, that the advantage may eventually be lost, because more Japanese are forsaking their traditional diet in favor of fast food and higher-fat diets.

Although cancer rates have steadily been rising in the United States, there's a lot we can do to reduce the risk—and most important is cutting the fat from our diet. In fact, the fat-cutting principles that help you fight cancer are the same as those that will reduce your risk for a lot of other diseases. In a nutshell, here's what experts recommend.

Strip the add-ons. Although breads and vegetables are naturally low in fat, the equation changes when you put fat on top—by spreading a thick layer of butter on bread, for instance, or topping a potato with gobs of sour cream. Make it a point to enjoy them *au naturel*. On your morning toast, spread just a thin layer of margarine—or, better yet, use only preserves. For potatoes, when you're craving add-ons like bacon or a fat dollop of regular sour cream, use these toppings sparingly. Better yet, replace all potato toppings with low-fat al-

SWEET AND SPICY CURRY DIP

To get the great taste and disease-fighting benefits of curry, bring out the low-fat chips and whip up this fabulous curry dip.

- ¼ cup fruit chutney
- 1 tablespoon curry powder
- 1 cup yogurt cheese (page 156)
- ⅛ teaspoon hot-pepper sauce

In a 1-quart saucepan over medium-low heat, stir together the chutney and curry powder for 1 minute to mix them well and remove some of the raw taste of the curry powder. Set aside for a few minutes to cool slightly.

In a small bowl, mix the yogurt cheese and hot-pepper sauce. Stir in the chutney mixture and blend well.

Makes about 1¼ cups.

Per tablespoon: 21 calories, 0.3 g. fat (14% of calories), 0.1 g. dietary fiber, 0 mg. cholesterol, 1 mg. sodium.

Spice for Life

Got a taste for fiery curry? Go ahead and indulge—your body will thank you for it.

In studies, scientists have found that curcumin decreases the growth of colon and breast cancers in lab animals. (Curcumin is the yellow pigment in turmeric, an ingredient in curry.) A possible explanation is that curcumin chemically alters carcinogens and flushes them from the body before they can cause problems.

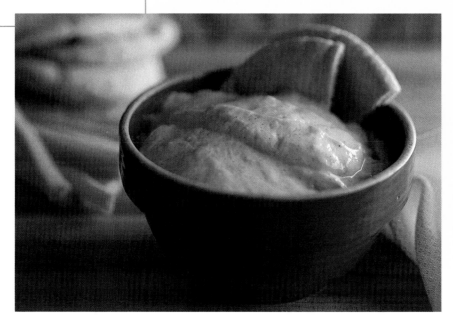

Sweet and Spicy Curry Dip served with pita bread

ternatives such as salsa, lemon juice or fat-free sour cream.

Ditch your steaks. Studies have shown that the saturated fats in red meats may significantly boost your risk of certain cancers. "Vegetarians have less prostate cancer than steak-lovers do," comments Neal Barnard, M.D., president of the Physicians Committee for Responsible Medicine in Washington, D.C., and author of *Food for Life*. There are also definite links between a red-meat diet and colon cancer.

When you do want meat, stick with lean cuts such as flank steak, and be sure to trim away all visible fat before cooking. Better yet, put the red meat aside and replace it with fish or skinless chicken or turkey.

Skim the risks. Whole milk may be less than wholesome. One eight-ounce glass contains nine grams of fat, most of them of the saturated variety. So switch to a low-fat or nonfat version. To make the transition more gradual—and palatable—first change over to 2 percent milk. Later, switch to 1 percent. Finally, when you're used to the taste of 1 percent milk, change to skim.

Cook the healthy way. Whether you're cooking green vegetables or fresh fish, a panful of cooking oil will cause your dinner to take on more of the slippery stuff than a supertanker. To reduce the fat and preserve the flavor, use healthier cooking methods such as baking, steaming, grilling or microwaving.

SCRUBBING THE RISK

There are several reasons why your colon would welcome carrots over cow any day. The dietary fiber in fruits, vegetables and whole grains isn't absorbed in the small intestine but instead is passed virtually unchanged into the colon. Once there, the fiber helps dilute the concentration of secondary bile acids (the acids that "soak up" unwanted waste) and any carcinogens that may be present. It also speeds their passage out

(continued on page 112)

A GARDEN IN A JAR

There's nothing fresher than soybean sprouts—they're still growing when you eat them!

Like most beans, soybeans and their sprouts are rich in isoflavones, protective plant compounds that may help tame the activity of cancer-causing enzymes in your body.

In laboratory studies at the University of Alabama, researchers found that tumors were less likely to develop in animals that were given soybeans as part of their daily diets. In addition, scientists have noted that in China and Japan, where soybeans are an important source of dietary protein, the rates of breast cancer are much lower than in the United States.

You don't have to drive to the supermarket or health food store to get the benefits of bean sprouts. Just by using a few simple sprouting tips, you can have your own cancer-fighting garden in a jar. Here's how to do it.

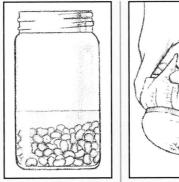 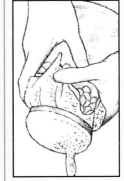 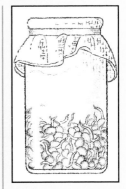

1. Soak the soybeans in a one-quart jar filled with slightly cool (70° to 80° F) water at a ratio of one part seeds to four parts water. The beans should soak for 8 to 12 hours in a dark, warm place.

After soaking the seeds, pour off the water. (You can reserve this fluid for soups or drinks, as it has a mild flavor and some nutrients.)

2. Rinse the soaked seeds and strain out all the water through a piece of cheesecloth secured at the top of the jar with a rubber band.

Keeping the cheesecloth on the jar, return it to the same warm, dark place. Sprouts should be rinsed and drained thoroughly twice a day. Any water that stays in the jar can cause mold.

3. You'll have fresh sprouts ready for eating within three to five days. But before you harvest the beans, allow them a quick peek at the sun for just a few hours. The sunlight will enable them to produce additional chlorophyll, increasing their nutritional value.

Any leftover sprouts can be stored in a closed container in the refrigerator.

Good Things That Grow on Trees

Many of us already begin our days with a sunny glass of orange juice. But if recent research is an indication of good things to come, we're going to be indulging a lot more often.

"Citrus fruits are packed with natural substances that may prevent cancer, reduce allergy symptoms and help protect the heart," says John Attaway, Ph.D., director of scientific research for the Florida Department of Citrus in Lake Alfred.

All the citrus fruits, from lemons and limes to kumquats, grapefruit and tangerines, are packed with vitamin C. As with the other antioxidants—like vitamin E and beta-carotene—vitamin C helps neutralize potentially cancer-causing molecules in the cells called free radicals. This is important because free radicals can attack vital components in your body.

In addition, studies show that vitamin C helps stimulate the immune sys-tem, making it more efficient at seeking out and destroying abnormal cells. When adequate vitamin C is present, the number of frontline infection fighters —such as T-cells and B-cells—increases.

Citrus fruits also contain a variety of cancer-fighting compounds called flavonoids, which include limonene, naringin, hesperidin, nobiletin and tangeretin.

The proof is in the testing. Tangeretin, for example, has been shown to help prevent cancer from invading normal cells, possibly preventing its growth and neutralizing the disease, says Dr. Attaway.

The benefits of vitamin C may be even more dramatic. In a survey of 11,348 adults, researchers at the University of California at Los Angeles focused on the 227 individuals who consumed over 750 milligrams of vitamin C daily—from foods as well as supplements.

During the ten-year period of the study, researchers found that the death rate among the group with the high vitamin C intake was 60 percent lower than among the people who had little or none of the vitamin in their diet.

In fact, studies have consistently shown that cancer rates are lower in people who eat the most fruit—a major source of vitamin C—says University of California professor Dr. Gladys Block.

"I do think the evidence is strong

ZEST FOR LIFE

For people who love citrus, there's nothing better than the zippy, nose-tingling smell of grated lemon or orange peel—that little twist of peel that chefs call the zest. Here's an added bonus: The same zest that's divine in angel cake and terrific in tea may also be fabulous for your health.

As we've mentioned, limonene, a flavoring agent that's extracted from the citrus peels, may be a potent protector against cancer. It appears to work in three ways: It stimulates enzymes that help remove excess estrogen from the body, it assists enzymes that break down potential carcinogens in your body, and it helps inhibit the growth of cancer cells before they spread.

Researchers have found that limonene can shrink mammary gland tumors in laboratory rats. And some laboratory studies have shown that compounds taken from tangerine peels—nobiletin and tangeretin— were able to inhibit cancer cell growth up to 88 percent in just five days.

More studies are needed, but it seems likely that people eating a high-citrus diet may glean at least some of the same benefits, researchers say.

STAYING ABOVE C LEVEL

Orange juice has a zingy, refreshing taste, and there's a lot to be said for the health benefits we get from its vitamin C. But when it comes to nutritional value, not all juices are created equal. Here are a few points to keep in mind.

Fresh is best. *The "fresh-squeezed" juice in the dairy case is also the freshest tasting. As you might expect, it also may boast the highest levels of vitamin C.*

Keep out the sunshine. *Many vitamins are sensitive to light and heat, which is why juice in bottles may contain less active vitamin C than juice in dark cartons.*

Read the labels. *While the manufacturing process destroys vitamin C, some juice concentrates are reconstituted by adding pulp and fresh juices— and with them an extra shot of vitamin C.*

HOW YOUR OJ MEASURES UP

Juice or Drink (1 cup)	Vitamin C (mg.)
Orange juice, raw, fresh	*124*
Orange juice, frozen concentrate, unsweetened, mixed with water	*97*
Orange juice, frozen concentrate, country-style (such as Minute Maid)	*96*
Orange juice, canned, unsweetened	*86*
Orange juice, frozen concentrate, homestyle (such as Tropicana)	*78*
Orange drink, with juice and pulp	*78*
Orange-flavored drink, with juice and pulp (such as Sunny Delight citrus punch)	*60*
Orange-flavored drink, 10% juice, canned (such as Hi-C)	*60*
Orange-flavored drink mix, powdered, 2 tablespoons mixed with water (such as Tang)	*60*
Orange punch with 100% fruit juices (such as Juicy Juice)	*60*

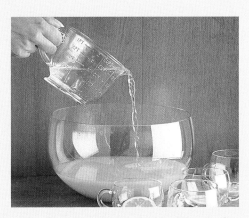

Citrus cooler is a punch that packs a punch . . . of vitamin C. For a festive touch, pour it into a punch bowl, adding club soda just before serving.

Citrus Cooler

With so much fruity variety out there, why limit yourself to OJ? This zingy punch will deliver virtually all of the protective nutrients you get in fruit and all of the taste. Each serving gives you about 70 milligrams of vitamin C.

- 1½   cups orange juice
- ½   cup grapefruit juice
- ¼   cup tangerine juice concentrate (see Note)
- 1   tablespoon lime juice
- 2   teaspoons sugar
- ¼   teaspoon almond extract
- ¼   teaspoon vanilla
- 2   cups club soda
- 4   lemon slices

Place the orange juice, grapefruit juice, tangerine juice, lime juice, sugar, almond extract and vanilla in the container of a blender. Cover and blend until well mixed.

Transfer to a large pitcher or punch bowl. Stir in the club soda. Serve over ice, garnished with the lemon slices.

Makes 4 servings.

Note: If tangerine concentrate is not available, you can substitute any other citrus juice.

Per serving: 75 calories, 0.2 g. fat (3% of calories), 0.9 g. dietary fiber, 0 mg. cholesterol, 26 mg. sodium.

enough for me to say that for prevention of *some* cancers, vitamin C probably makes a difference," she says.

Orange juice always contains vitamin C, though amounts may vary depending on how the juice is prepared and stored (see above). Most orange-flavored drinks and punches also have vitamin C, though in lower amounts.

Your body absorbs almost 100 percent of the first 30 to 60 milligrams of vitamin C that you consume each day. Above that, the percentage of absorption gradually declines. When there is excess vitamin C in your bloodstream, it's either absorbed by various tissues—including the lungs, kidneys and liver—or excreted in the urine.

of the body—and out of harm's way.

"When you eat more fiber, you tend to have a fast passage time of the feces through the bowel. Therefore, the surface of the bowel is not exposed—or at least does not have a long exposure—to any carcinogens that may be there," explains Thomas Jefferson Hospital's Dr. Mansfield.

Also, dietary fiber changes the acidity of the bowel, making it less hospitable to bacteria that may promote changes that can lead to colon cancer, says Dr. Trock.

When researchers analyzed more than 37 studies involving more than 10,000 people, they found that those who ate the most fiber-rich foods were able to substantially lower their colon cancer risk—by as much as 40 percent, in some cases.

MEDICINE IN ITS OWN RIGHT

For years, experts suspected that increasing fiber intake was just another way to reduce fat, since most high-fiber diets are naturally low in fat. But telltale research changed their minds.

In Finland, overall fat consumption equals or exceeds that of most industrialized nations. You would expect to find a high rate of colon cancer there. But the Finns also eat a lot of whole-grain, high-fiber foods. The result? They have about one-third our risk for colon cancer.

While some studies suggest that the fiber found in wheat bran and rye bran may be most effective, "it's counterproductive to split hairs," says Dr. Trock. "The most important thing the public can do is increase its overall intake of fresh fruits and vegetables and grains from a variety of natural food sources."

Experts recommend that we eat up to 35 grams of fiber every day. Having a bowl of oatmeal or other high-fiber cereal in the morning will start the day right with about 4 grams of fiber. Add to that a few slices of whole-wheat bread or toast (about 1 gram each) and several pieces of fruit (an apple provides 3 grams, while five ounces of figs deliver 5

PUNGENT PROTECTION

Garlic has long been disparaged as the "stinking rose," but research suggests it may soon be better known for promoting the bloom of health.

When you eat garlic, it releases a powerful compound called allicin. Allicin has been shown to lower blood pressure and cholesterol and possibly to help reduce the risk for developing cancer.

Researchers in China have noted that in areas where garlic consumption is high (about ¾ of an ounce per day), the rate of stomach cancer is only one-tenth as high as in areas where consumption is low. Closer to home, researchers from the National Cancer Institute report that liberal consumption of garlic and onions has been associated with a decreased incidence of colorectal cancer.

Researchers aren't sure how garlic protects. According to John A. Milner, Ph.D., professor of nutrition and head of the Department of Nutrition at Pennsylvania State University in University Park, it may somehow block the formation of cancer-causing compounds or possibly limit their ability to cause tumors.

In its raw state, garlic can be a little too potent for most people. Roasting, however, helps tone down its forceful flavor, bringing out a sweeter, nuttier taste.

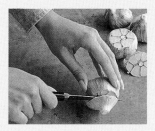

1. Cut the tops off the garlic heads and arrange them snugly in a small baking dish.

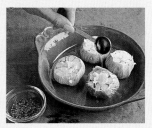

2. Moisten the heads with a little olive oil. Then cover and bake at 300° for half an hour.

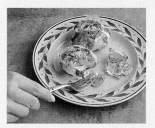

3. Uncover and bake for one hour, or until tender. The husk of the garlic should be golden brown.

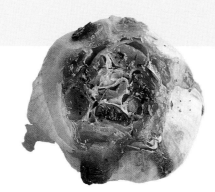

grams). Add it up, and you'll see you're already halfway there.

Other good fiber sources include most fruits, vegetables, beans, pastas and whole grains. Let your taste buds be your guide. "The main thing is, a high-fiber diet provides a lot of fiber and a lot of micronutrients, and it's low in fat," says Dr. Trock. "So let's not worry about which piece of it prevents cancer."

FRUITS, GREENS AND OTHER HEALTHY THINGS

Since 1971, more than 175 published studies have looked at the relationship between cancer and fruits and vegetables, as well as some of the nutrients they contain.

According to Gladys Block, Ph.D., professor of public health at the University of California, Berkeley, School of Public Health, the evidence is "extraordinarily consistent" that as our intake of these foods goes up, our cancer risks go down.

Nature's bounty protects on several fronts. Fruits and vegetables are packed with fiber, and they're low in fat—which are two very potent weapons in the cancer wars. Nutrients in some fruits are thought to enhance the anti-cancer activity of naturally occurring enzymes in the body.

Also, many fruits and vegetables contain one or more of the antioxidants such as vitamins E and C and beta-carotene and bioflavonoids, which gobble up harmful oxygen molecules in the cells before they cause damage that might lead to cancer.

"There could be protective nutrients that we don't even recognize yet," says Dr. Mansfield. "What we can say is that beta-carotene and some of the other antioxidants have been the high rankers in preventing some types of cancer."

THE FRIDGE THAT FOILED CANCER

In the days before refrigeration and long-distance transportation, many people were unable to enjoy fresh fruits and produce year-round—and at least part of their diet consisted of smoked and salted foods. And when meats spoiled, they carried bacteria that contributed to stomach cancer. Also, in order to prevent spoilage, foods were treated with preservatives containing nitrates. In our bodies, nitrates are chemically changed into nitrites, then to nitrosamines—and nitrosamines are the carcinogens that cause stomach cancer. Not surprisingly, then, stomach cancer was quite common in the days when people ate large amounts of smoked and salted preserved foods.

In the modern supermarket, however, fresh foods are always available. And guess what? The incidence of stomach cancer has gone down steadily over the past 30 to 40 years.

But with less than 10 percent of Americans actually getting the five servings of fruits and vegetables recommended by the NCI, many of us are not taking advantage of the modern fresh food supply.

While five servings a day may seem like a lot, it adds up quickly, says Dr. Block. "It's not as hard as it sounds to get five servings in," she says. "A glass of fruit juice at breakfast, a piece of fruit with lunch, another as a snack and two vegetables with dinner will do it."

But which nutrients are the most important? For good health, all are essential, but here's what experts recommend for boosting your cancer-prevention plan.

BOOSTING YOUR C

Dr. Block looked at dozens of studies that estimated people's intake of vitamin C and examined how often they got cancer. Out of 46 population studies, she found that 33 gave strong evidence that the people whose diets contained the most vitamin C had the lowest risk of cancer.

"The evidence for a protective effect of vitamin C was especially strong in cancer of the mouth, larynx, esophagus, stomach, pancreas, rectum and uterine cervix," she says. "And there is in-

POLLUTION PROTECTION

You don't have to be jammed in rush-hour traffic on an L.A. freeway to know that fresh air isn't what it used to be. Every minute of every day we're breathing in car exhaust, second-hand cigarette smoke and many other types of pollution. With every breath, we inhale a vast array of toxins that can lead to cancer.

We can't always change the air we breathe, but we can cut the risks—by eating right. Past research has shown that people who get high levels of key nutrients—among them vitamins C and E and beta-carotene—can help ward off a variety of cancers caused by environmental hazards.

Because these nutrients have so much going for them, some experts now advise that people who have a high risk for cancer—smokers, for example—should make a special effort to up their intake of all fruits and vegetables. Ranked high on the list of recommended vegetables are those that are stocked with beta-carotene, such as kale, broccoli, squash and spinach.

The Cruciferous Connection

When it comes to delivering a powerful, cancer-pounding punch, cruciferous vegetables are ferocious fighters.

Cabbage, broccoli, cauliflower and brussels sprouts may look like common, everyday garden vegetables, but like other crucifers (the name is a reference to their cross-shaped leaf formations), they contain a number of powerful compounds that can help cross out the cancer risk.

Studies have shown that the compound called sulforaphane, for example, can help boost the body's production of protective enzymes that help detoxify and remove carcinogens from the body before they cause problems.

Cruciferous vegetables also contain a group of protective compounds called indoles, which accelerate the rate at which estrogen can be "neutralized" by the body. (And this is important in fighting breast cancer—as shown on pages 106 and 107.)

In a review of 137 studies, researchers at the University of Minnesota School of Public Health in Minneapolis found that eating more fruits and vegetables was consistently linked to a reduced risk of cancer.

In addition, studies have shown that

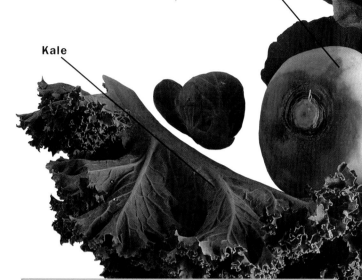

Turnip

Kale

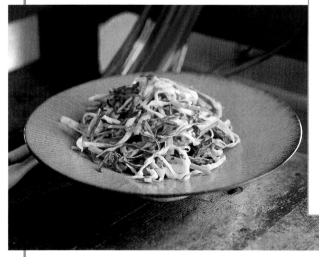

RAW SLAW TO RELISH

Here's a great way to get the benefits of a star crucifer—cabbage—in a delicious side dish. Though restaurant coleslaw may be overloaded with fat and salt because of mayonnaise and other ingredients, the recipe below is tailored for a low-fat menu. If you have a food processor to slice up the cabbage, it takes just a few minutes to make.

    3   cups thinly sliced red cabbage
    2½ cups thinly sliced green cabbage
    1   large carrot, julienned
    3   scallions, julienned
    ¼   cup lemon juice
    ¼   cup nonfat mayonnaise
    1   clove garlic, minced
    ½   teaspoon grated fresh ginger
    2   tablespoons snipped chives

Combine the red cabbage, green cabbage, carrots and scallions in a large bowl.

In another bowl, mix the lemon juice, mayonnaise, garlic and ginger. Pour over the cabbage and toss well. Sprinkle with the chives.

Makes 6 servings.

Per serving: 42 calories, 0.2 g. fat (4% of calories), 2 g. dietary fiber, 0 mg. cholesterol, 83 mg. sodium.

ACCENT ON TASTE

While cruciferous vegetables have powerful nutrients, they also have powerful tastes. Indeed, if you've ever cooked cabbage or cauliflower with the windows closed, you know these vegetables possess some of the strongest flavors—and smells—in the vegetable kingdom.

Here are two quick ways to enjoy the benefits of crucifers in a minimum of cooking time.

■ *Heat a tablespoon of olive oil in a wok or large saucepan. Add coarsely chopped greens such as kale, dandelion or mustard, and cook only until they wilt. Season with crushed garlic and red pepper and serve.*

■ *Steam two cups of your favorite crucifer until crunchy-tender. Add the vegetables to one pound of cooked pasta, along with a sprinkle of Parmesan cheese and a drizzle of olive oil. Toss and serve.*

Radishes

Brussels Sprouts

Chinese Cabbage (Bok Choy)

Kohlrabi

women who eat cruciferous vegetables at least four times a week have lower blood levels of estradiol, the form of estrogen associated with breast cancer, says Leon Bradlow, Ph.D., director of biomedical endocrinology at the Strang-Cornell Cancer Research Laboratory in New York City.

"The effect of eating cruciferous vegetables is quite clear," he says. "Within about a week of starting a test diet that included servings of these vegetables, the women in our study had a measurable drop in this 'bad' estrogen in their blood."

As an added benefit, the cruciferous family is a large one, including not only cabbage and broccoli but also kale, kohlrabi and mustard greens. Your taste buds will never get bored.

It's important, however, to cook them with care. In one study, Canadian researchers found that prolonged cooking could reduce the amount of available cancer-fighting indoles by as much as 50 percent.

For the best of both worlds—getting the cancer-fighting nutrients of crucifers plus the great taste—cook them only until they're tender, experts say. You may even enjoy crunching them raw.

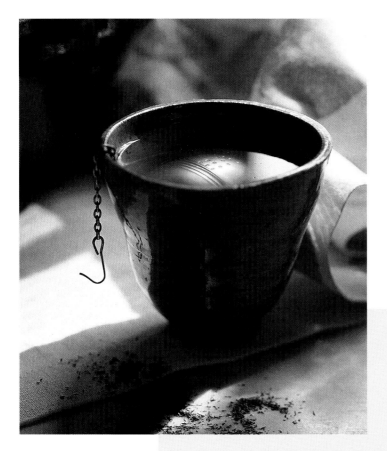

You can find green tea at your local health food store or Asian market. Use one to two tablespoons of dried tea per cup of boiling water and steep to taste.

PROTECTION BREWING

Researchers have been puzzled by the fact that people in Japan have a lower rate of lung cancer than Americans. The reason, some experts say, is green tea: We drink very little of it, and they drink a lot.

Green tea is perhaps the most popular beverage in Asia. It's not uncommon for people to drink up to ten small cups a day. Researchers speculate that there are substances in green tea that may help block the formation of cancer-causing compounds and also may "trap" carcinogens before they cause damage.

In a study at the National Cancer Research Institute in Tokyo, mice given a chemical extracted from green tea were far less likely to develop cancer of the digestive tract than animals not given protection. In another study, this one at Rutgers University in New Brunswick, New Jersey, mice given green tea for ten days developed, on average, half as many tumors as those given only water.

creasing evidence of a role in preventing lung cancer."

Vitamin C is an antioxidant, which means it helps mop up those damaging oxygen molecules in the cells called free radicals—the same free radicals that are to blame for so many of the aging processes in our bodies. These molecules, despite being a normal part of the body's metabolism, can eventually damage genetic material, which in turn can lead to cancer.

There's also evidence that vitamin C may prevent or delay the growth of tumors that are triggered by high levels of hormones such as estrogen, according to Joachim G. Liehr, Ph.D., professor of pharmacology at the University of Texas Medical Branch at Galveston. Vitamin C also stimulates the immune system so that it fights off invaders more efficiently.

The Daily Value (DV) for vitamin C is 60 milligrams. Most doctors agree that this is an adequate amount for overall health. But they also note that for cancer prevention, larger amounts may be needed. By eating just one orange a day, you will get the minimum requirement. You can boost that amount with other foods such as grapefruit, cantaloupe, strawberries and fruit juices, which are also high in vitamin C.

BANKING ON BETA-CAROTENE

This is one of those situations where nature has accomplished some artful color-coding, and we're the beneficiaries. The telltale colors are dark green, yellow and orange, and they're found in fruits and vegetables. The colors are the giveaway that beta-carotene is present in these foods.

Beta-carotene is one of the compounds that gives plants their color. When humans consume this powerful nutrient, it has been shown to help prevent a host of different cancers, including those of the lung, breast and cervix.

It was formerly thought that the principal benefit of beta-carotene was that the body could convert it to vitamin A on an as-needed basis. More recent findings have shown that as an antioxidant, beta-carotene seems to work its magic without undergoing the transformation into vitamin A. Moreover, while few studies point to an association between cancer protection and high levels of vitamin A in the body, research consistently demonstrates that there is a significant link between high levels of beta-carotene and lower rates of certain cancers.

In a study at the University of Washington in Seattle, researchers found that women who consumed the largest amounts of dark green and yellow vegetables (high in beta-carotene) were able to reduce their risk of cervical cancer by 60 percent.

In another study, researchers at the University of Utah School of Medicine in Salt Lake City compared the diets of 85 women with ovarian tumors with the diets of 492 healthy women. They found that the women who ate the most foods rich in beta-carotene and related carotenoids—like alpha- and gamma-carotene—were half as likely to get ovarian cancer as those who ate the least. (Carotenoid-rich foods include carrots, sweet potatoes, acorn squash, spinach and cantaloupe.)

This nutrient's protective abilities may extend to cancer of the lung, as well. In a Swiss study of 2,974 men, researchers found that those with low blood levels of beta-carotene had a significantly higher risk of death from lung cancer.

These findings led the researchers to "strongly encourage a higher intake of dietary carotenoids and carotene-containing supplements as a preventive measure against cancer."

Although the government has not yet established a DV for any of the carotenoids, you can probably get an adequate amount of these important nutrients if you follow the dietary guidelines that are recommended by the NCI, says epidemiologist Dr. Potischman. "If you really strive toward eating more than five servings of a variety of fruits and vegetables a day, then you're right on target," she says.

EXTENDING YOUR E

Like beta-carotene and vitamin C, vitamin E is an antioxidant vitamin that will help scavenge harmful free radicals from your cells before they can cause damage.

According to an NCI study, people taking vitamin E supplements were able to cut in half their risk of contracting cancer of the mouth or throat. And in a five-year study of 35,215 women, researchers at the University of Minnesota in Minneapolis found that those who developed colon cancer were the ones who got the smallest amounts of vitamin E.

"Vitamin E has a very strong ability to protect cell membranes against cell destruction," says study leader Roberd Bostick, M.D., Ph.D., assistant professor of epidemiology at the university. "Strong cell membranes may be particularly important in the colon because the bacteria there produce a lot of free radicals"—those unstable molecules that can lead to tumors.

You may have to take extra steps to get the protective benefits of vitamin E. Just as extra vitamin E is needed to help protect cells from certain aging processes, its anti-cancer benefits may kick in only at doses higher than the DV. Although the DV for vitamin E is 30 international units, Dr. Bostick's study showed protective benefits only at amounts greater than 36 international units.

You can get enough vitamin E from your diet alone, although you may have to work at it. The best sources of vitamin E are, unfortunately, also high in fat. They include sunflower oil, safflower oil and almond oil. You can also get some vitamin E, although in much smaller amounts, from foods such as apples, toasted wheat germ and black currants.

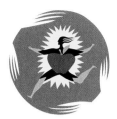

BREAKTHROUGHS IN HEALING

1 9 9 0

A study of over 88,000 women by Walter C. Willett, M.D., and others at Harvard Medical School concludes that people who eat foods high in animal fat have a significantly greater risk of colon cancer.

1 9 9 1

Reviewing 16 years of studies on vitamin E, researchers conclude that adequate levels of the vitamin reduce the incidence of certain cancers.

1 9 9 2

A review of 156 scientific studies that looked at the relationship between diet and cancer finds "extraordinarily consistent scientific evidence" supporting the protective effect of certain foods. For the first time, evidence seems conclusive that people whose diets are rich in fruits and vegetables are less likely to get a wide variety of cancers.

1 9 9 4

Researchers at Johns Hopkins University in Baltimore provide dramatic support for the theory that sulforaphane—found in broccoli—helps protect animals against cancer. When laboratory animals are treated with sulforaphane, far fewer animals develop tumors.

Supercharge Your Immune System

Every minute of every day, a feeding frenzy takes place within your body. Invading bacteria from outside sources such as food, air and water make their way through the bloodstream, trying to gang up on cells to control them. Luckily, your internal army of fighting cells is there to keep the peace. Among them are macrophages (shown in photo at right), bacteria-eating defenders that are produced in bone marrow and kill invading bacteria with a powerful chemical. Macrophages literally eat the invaders one by one, digesting them and turning them into energy.

A number of hormonelike sub-

One innocent "ah-choo!" from a co-worker, and a drifting cloud of viruses floats through the air. Bacteria and fungi clandestinely attack our bodies through our noses, mouths or skin. Various parasites that we consume in food and water harm our intestinal tract, lungs, liver or brain. Even pollutants and toxins in air and water weaken our immunity and trigger life-threatening diseases.

Any one of these microscopic menaces can cause an infection or trigger a disease. Yet each day our bodies must do battle with untold billions of them—over one million bacteria can live on a single inch of freshly washed skin.

A strong immune system can not only wipe out these invaders before they can cause illness but can also help prevent and control serious conditions like cancer. There's even research that indicates that a strong immune system can delay the onset of AIDS in those infected with HIV.

The problem is, immunity tends to weaken with each passing year. "As you age and reach your fifties and sixties, your immune system changes," says Ronald Watson, Ph.D., research professor at the University of Arizona College of Medicine in Tucson. "Your infection-fighting cells don't function as well, placing you at greater risk for infection and cancer."

Unseen, your body fights constant battles with its invaders. "I hate to use military terminology, but it's really war going on inside your body between these infectors and your immune system," adds Terry Phillips, Ph.D., D.Sc., director of the immunogenetics and the immunochemistry laboratories at George Washington University Medical Center in Washington, D.C., and co-author of *Winning the War Within: Understanding, Protecting and Building Your Body's Immunity*. "If you think of your body as being a country, the immune system is the army—attacking these invaders to keep the peace."

And as Napoleon said, "An army marches on its stomach." Or at least, scientists may add, the right diet can keep it strong.

"The immune system is like every other system in the human body: It requires a healthy diet in order to function properly," says Dr. Phillips. "And certain nutrients have been shown to boost your immune system's response and make you more resistant to disease. Besides that, the right diet gives you the energy you need so you can exercise—which also keeps immunity strong—and ensures you get the proper sleep so your immune system gets a chance to repair itself."

Benign, slow-moving cells that guard your body, macrophages reach out and engulf invading bacteria. Here, a large, brownish-colored macrophage traps Escherichia coli *bacteria (shown in blue). As it ingests the bacteria, the macrophage will break down and destroy the invading cells with powerful chemicals.*

stances called macrophage activating factors (MAF) can stimulate the macrophages, inducing them to change shape and size—and to attack invaders. When activated, the macrophage increases in size, produces granular-shaped bumps on its surface and begins to spread out with long, elastic "feet" called pseudopods.

Unfortunately, as you age, macrophages and other defenders called T-cells tend to be less effective at defending your body against bacteria and other invaders. You can help offset this weakening of the immune system by eating a low-fat diet rich in certain key nutrients—among them vitamin B_6, the antioxidant vitamins C and E and beta-carotene, and minerals like zinc, copper, selenium, iron and magnesium.

MEET YOUR PROTECTOR

Food is needed for the care and feeding of the billions of new cells produced in your body each day. Since most of these cells live only a few days, they constantly need to be replaced. Among these cells are the warriors that comprise your immune system. These guardians of your body protect you from what are generally called antigens—the term used for anything thought to be an invader, such as viruses, bacteria, dust or chemicals. Your body protectors include:

■ Antibodies. These Y-shaped protein molecules rush to the infection site, neutralizing the enemy with a chemical or tagging it for attack by other cells.

■ Killer T-cells. These cells are so named because they mature in the thymus, a lymph gland that sits be-

hind the breastbone. Killer T-cells do the dirty work—specializing in killing cells that have been invaded by foreign organisms such as viruses, bacteria and other attackers. They also destroy cells that have become cancerous.

■ Helper T-cells. These do-gooders actually identify the antigen and then call in the reinforcements—which are usually killer T-cells.

■ Suppressor T-cells. These specialized cells assist helper cells in mobilizing the fighting force. But their main job is to call off the troops once the infection has been conquered.

■ B-cells. These brutes are like arms dealers. Formed in bone marrow, they deploy the weapons—the powerful chemicals used by your antibodies and your T-cells to destroy the enemy. The B-cells also carry the

IMMUNITY IN A PILL

As we age, our immune system tends to function less efficiently, making us more prone to disease. While the best way to keep immunity strong is with a diet that's rich in infection-fighting vitamins and minerals—like those found in fruits and vegetables—the reality is that we often don't have the time or appetite to eat the recommended five or more servings a week.

But that doesn't mean that you're destined to have a tarnished immune system in your golden years, thanks to a multivitamin supplement that's been proven to bolster the immune system. Researchers gave healthy people between the ages of 66 and 86 this immunity-boosting supplement with the nutrients listed in the table at right, while another group of seniors was given a placebo (blank pill). After one year, the researchers noted that the group taking the supplement got half the number of infection-related illnesses as the group taking the placebo.

Of course, supplements shouldn't be used as replacements for healthy eating. But if you're going to take a multivitamin, try to get one that is similar to this immunity-boosting formula.

"memory" of previous battles with specific antigens. Essentially, they keep records of previous battles so that any repeat invasion by a former foe can be immediately countered. When the T-cells are called up as reinforcements, the B-cells often enter the fray with them.

■ Macrophages. These are big cells that move slowly through the bloodstream, looking for any signs of trouble. When they find an antigen, they turn into monstrous gluttons that engulf and eat it. Macrophages also summon helper T-cells to the scene.

■ Neutrophils. These are the search-and-destroy team of the immune system. These cells are faster moving than macrophages, which ooze amoeba-like through cells in your blood vessels. A neutrophil flows around its prey, enveloping it and then destroying it with enzymes.

It's a highly specialized system, with each cell having a specific role. But you're the one who feeds the troops. And when you eat the right diet, you help them do their job.

FORMULA FOR A SUPER SUPPLEMENT

The amounts of some of the nutrients in this daily supplement—thiamin, vitamins B$_6$ and C and copper—are moderately higher than the Daily Value. The supplement also contains selenium, calcium, magnesium and other nutrients that help boost immunity.

NUTRIENT	AMOUNT
Vitamin A	400 RE
Thiamin	2.2 mg
Riboflavin	1.5 mg.
Niacin	16 mg.
Folate	400 mcg.
Vitamin B$_6$	3 mg.
Vitamin B$_{12}$	4 mcg.
Vitamin C	80 mg.
Vitamin D	4 mcg.
Vitamin E	44 mg.
Beta-carotene	16 mg.
Calcium	200 mg.
Copper	1.4 mg.
Iodine	0.2 mg.
Iron	16 mg.
Magnesium	100 mg.
Selenium	2 mcg.
Zinc	14 mg.

ANTIOXIDANTS: YOUR HOTSHOT IMMUNE BOOSTERS

Leading the "Most Wanted" list of immunity-boosting vitamins are the "big three" antioxidants—vitamins C and E and beta-carotene.

These antioxidants help build immunity for the same reasons they protect against cancer and keep you looking and feeling younger.

"An antioxidant is anything that scavenges free radicals and protects against oxidative damage," says Harinder Garewal, M.D., Ph.D., assistant director of cancer prevention and control at the Veterans Administration Hospital and the Arizona Cancer Center, both in Tucson, who pioneered the study of beta-carotene as a possible way of decreasing cancer risk. "There are several antioxidant vitamins, but the interest in these three, I suppose, stems from the fact that they are abundant in so many foods and are essentially nontoxic, even in moderately large doses."

In a review of more than 200 studies that were conducted over a 20-year period, the Alliance for Aging Research—a Washington, D.C.–based public health organization—concluded that vitamins C and E and beta-carotene do help to squelch free radicals. While scientific researchers have not agreed on specific recommendations, they do suggest some ways that you can get more antioxidant vitamins in your food. Here's how.

Seek out citrus. "There's been more study on vitamin C than anything else, which may explain why it's been shown to do more than just about any other vitamin," says Dr. Phillips. "We know it affects the thymus and lymph glands, helps produce more cells and stimulates tumor-attack cells—all factors in boosting immunity. It also is supposed to produce antibody cells. Citrus fruits like oranges and grapefruit are among the best sources of vitamin C."

Bag some tropical fruits. If you're snacking on fruit, you'll also get vitamin C in lesser-known fruits like guavas, papaya and kiwi fruit. In fact, the so-called tropical fruits can contain twice as much vitamin C as an orange. While they're not always available at your local supermarket, you should grab them when you see them. You'll not only get that extra vitamin C boost, you'll also get—if you haven't had them before—an intriguing surprise for your taste buds. Other good sources, when they're in season, are cherries, black currants and honeydew melon.

Get E in nuts and seeds. Almonds, other nuts and sunflower seeds are among the best food sources of vitamin E. Actually, you'll get more vitamin E from cooking oils than anything else, but easy does it: Even "healthy" oils get all their calories from fat and can add extra pounds.

"Vitamin E is an inhibitor of free radicals, and it's also supposed to be good for red blood cells," says Dr. Phillips. "It also helps boost immunity by stimulating B- and T-cells."

Squash disease—with squash. The best sources of beta-carotene are fruits and vegetables that have an orange or yellow color, such as squash, pumpkin, mangoes and carrots, as well as green leafy vegetables such as spinach and kale.

"Beta-carotene stimulates the natural killer cells' activity and has an overall positive effect on immunity," says Dr. Garewal.

ONE SECRET FOR A HEALTHY OLD AGE: VITAMIN B$_6$

If you want to live to a healthy old age—or just want to stay healthy as you age—make sure you eat plenty of bananas, potatoes, turkey white meat and chick-peas. These foods are rich in vitamin B$_6$, which has long been known to stimulate the activity of T-cells—your immune system's main fighting force against invading bacteria and viruses.

What hasn't been known, however, is why immunity seems to weaken as you age. One possible explanation: "Elderly people seem to metabolize B$_6$ less effectively than younger people," says Simin Nibbin Meydani, Ph.D., of the U.S. Department of Agriculture Human Nutrition Research Center on Aging at Tufts University in Boston. "This could possibly lead to a B$_6$ deficiency, and such a deficiency can hurt immunity because of weakened T-cell activity."

But the more B$_6$ you consume from foods, the more "alert" your T-cells become, making you more resistant to possible infection. Usually you can get enough vitamin B$_6$ from food sources. (If you take a supplement, it should only be under a doctor's supervision, since high doses of supplemental vitamin B$_6$ have been known to cause nerve damage.)

And what's enough? "Shoot for the Daily Value of two milligrams a day—or even a little more," says Dr. Meydani. That's the amount you'd find in three bananas or about nine ounces of fresh tuna or three potatoes.

Minerals: An Immunity-Boosting Gold Mine

Some essential, hard-hitting minerals can give you the protection you need against infections and disease—particularly as you age. What's more, a little goes a long way. "Usually, there's no need to take supplements for these minerals," says Dr. Ananda Prasad, a zinc researcher at Wayne State University School of Medicine. "A good diet is usually enough to supply you with what you need." The targets on these pages show many of the foods that help keep your immunity strong by contributing minerals.

Zinc, for example, is a proven immunity booster that helps build killer T-cells, helper T-cells and suppressor T-cells. Since these are the cells that identify antigens and rush to kill infected or cancerous cells, zinc is an essential mineral. It helps the defenders do their defense work.

Iron plays a role in carrying oxygen to all cells—including immune cells that engulf invading bacteria and kill them with a deadly chemical. If you have low levels of iron, you might be more susceptible to bacterial infections, especially in your intestinal tract. Low iron can also make you more prone to viruses, since defenses are weakened by lack of this mineral.

Copper helps keep the immune system working hard when it's fighting infection. A deficiency in copper may lead to a lower white blood cell count and less resistance to infections. And if you don't have enough copper, cells that kill dangerous bacteria or viruses may become less active.

Selenium activates the infection-fighting troops in your immune system's army and prevents oxidative damage to cells. It also boosts the immune system function of vitamin E and prevents cancerous tumors.

Magnesium is a mineral that helps make infection-fighting white blood cells. Fall short on this nutrient and your immune system can become overstimulated and aggressive, with immune cells attacking and damaging the body.

So have a look at these targets and put some of these high-mineral foods on your next shopping list. If you aim for the foods near the bull's-eyes, you'll be doing your infection fighters a favor.

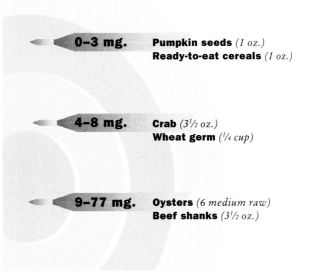

0–3 mg.   **Pumpkin seeds** *(1 oz.)*
Ready-to-eat cereals *(1 oz.)*

4–8 mg.   **Crab** *(3½ oz.)*
Wheat germ *(¼ cup)*

9–77 mg.   **Oysters** *(6 medium raw)*
Beef shanks *(3½ oz.)*

ZINC

The Daily Value for zinc is 15 milligrams for adults, but some nutritionists say that premenopausal women need up to 20 milligrams per day. That requirement falls back to 15 milligrams daily after menopause. Zinc is lost during sweating and every time a man ejaculates. Iron also interferes with zinc absorption.

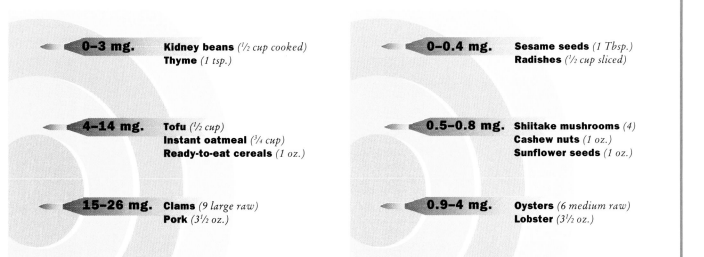

0–3 mg.	Kidney beans *(½ cup cooked)* Thyme *(1 tsp.)*
4–14 mg.	Tofu *(½ cup)* Instant oatmeal *(¾ cup)* Ready-to-eat cereals *(1 oz.)*
15–26 mg.	Clams *(9 large raw)* Pork *(3½ oz.)*

0–0.4 mg.	Sesame seeds *(1 Tbsp.)* Radishes *(½ cup sliced)*
0.5–0.8 mg.	Shiitake mushrooms *(4)* Cashew nuts *(1 oz.)* Sunflower seeds *(1 oz.)*
0.9–4 mg.	Oysters *(6 medium raw)* Lobster *(3½ oz.)*

IRON

The Daily Value for iron has been set at 18 milligrams per day for both men and women. Although meat is often thought of as the primary source of iron, there's also abundant iron in beans, nuts, seeds and tofu.

COPPER

Veal and lamb liver are good sources of copper, but these organ meats are high in cholesterol. Next best are oysters. At the first sign of a cold, doctors say, it might be wise to increase copper intake slightly.

0–6 mcg.	Egg *(1)* Cheddar cheese *(1 oz.)*
7–30 mcg.	Chicken breast *(3½ oz.)* English muffin *(1)* Mushrooms *(3½ oz. raw)*
31–76 mcg.	Salmon *(3½ oz.)* French bread *(3 pc.)*

4–9 mg.	Instant tea *(1 tsp. powder in 1 cup water)* Oregano *(1 tsp.)* Coffee *(6 oz.—8.9 mg.)*
10–40 mg.	Ready-to-eat cereals *(1 oz.)* Cowpeas *(½ cup cooked)*
41–102 mg.	Sesame seeds *(1 oz. dry roasted)* Rice bran *(2 Tbsp.)*

SELENIUM

Though there is no Daily Value for selenium, many nutritionists recommend that you get at least 70 micrograms every day—the amount you'd get from half a tuna sandwich. Selenium is found in virtually every food, with the highest amounts coming from fish, shellfish and whole grains.

MAGNESIUM

Both men and women need about 400 milligrams a day of magnesium. You'd get that from a couple of handfuls of sesame seeds. Certain prescription drugs can deplete magnesium stores, so check with your doctor about this if you're taking long-term medication. Drinking alcohol can also deplete magnesium.

THE ZINC LINK: UNDERRATED BUT ESSENTIAL

"You hear a lot about the antioxidant vitamins, which protect against damage done by oxidation—a process that can weaken immunity," says Dr. Phillips. "But they're only part of the story. In fact, there are other nutrients that may be just as important—or even more so—in keeping immunity strong."

Leading the list is zinc, an often overlooked and underappreciated mineral best known for helping to heal wounds and build tissues. "It may also be the single most important key to a healthy immune system," says Dr. Phillips.

Since it helps build T-cells, zinc is a front-line defender in a strong immune system. Studies show that people deficient in zinc are more prone to infection and overall immunity weakness. Research has also found that people with immune system problems may be able to correct such problems if they take zinc supplements, according to zinc researcher Ananda Prasad, M.D., Ph.D., professor of medicine at Wayne State University School of Medicine in Detroit. But even if you do not have a mineral deficiency problem, it does your body good to make sure it has an adequate zinc supply. Among the foods that are high in zinc and can help you be more resistant to disease are meat and potatoes.

For both men and women, the recommended level, or Daily Value, for zinc is 15 milligrams per day. Women, however, should get up to 20 milligrams per day during their childbearing years, according to Dr. Prasad. "Unfortunately, most people only get about half that amount—between 8 and 10 milligrams," says Dr. Prasad. If you get a lot of fiber in your diet and very little meat, you may have a zinc deficit, according to Dr. Prasad. (Your doctor will be able to tell you if there's a problem.) But for many other health conditions—such as high cholesterol and high blood pressure—a high-fiber, low-fat diet is recommended. So what tactics can you

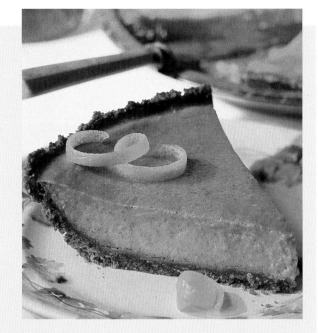

Here's a low-fat version of the classic Thanksgiving dessert. Garnish it with a sliver of orange peel instead of serving it with the usual whipped cream.

BETA-BETTERING PUMPKIN PIE

Improve your immunity any time of year with a slice of pumpkin pie—a bountiful source of beta-carotene. This recipe is low in fat and cholesterol.

1	cup graham cracker crumbs
2	tablespoons canola oil
1	cup fat-free egg substitute
1	cup evaporated skim milk
1	cup canned pumpkin
½	cup honey
1	teaspoon ground cinnamon
¼	teaspoon ground apple pie spice
⅛	teaspoon ground cloves

In a small bowl, mix the crumbs and oil. Coat a 9" pie plate with no-stick spray. Press the crumb mixture evenly into the bottom and up the sides of the pan.

Bake the crust at 350° for 7 minutes. Let cool on a wire rack while you prepare the filling.

In a medium bowl, whisk together the egg substitute, milk, pumpkin, honey, cinnamon, apple pie spice and cloves. Pour into the prepared crust. Bake for 40 minutes or until the center of the filling doesn't jiggle when you gently shake the pan. Cool completely before cutting.

Makes 8 servings

Per serving: 198 calories, 4.4 g. fat (20% of calories), 0.9 g. dietary fiber, 1 mg. cholesterol, 145 mg. sodium.

Mushrooms Show Their Magic

It's been over 2,000 years since Chinese herbalists first started using mushrooms to cure disease. Now Western doctors are discovering that this free-growing fungus may also help prevent it.

Several types of mushrooms—including shiitake and reishi—contain compounds called polysaccharides that boost immunity. Reishi mushrooms have also been shown to inhibit the development of cancer cells and reduce their number. In studies at the University of Texas Health Science Center in San Antonio, for example, reishi extracts were shown to have a significant anti-inflammatory effect. Other studies show that a diet rich in these mushrooms may help lessen problems associated with a variety of diseases, ranging from arthritis to chronic fatigue syndrome.

WHERE TO BUY IMMUNITY-BOOSTERS

Shiitake mushrooms, usually sold in dried form, are known for their firm texture and intense smoky flavor. If you get these mushrooms in dried form rather than fresh, they're easy to soften up for slicing: Simply soak them in boiling water for 15 to 20 minutes, until they're soft, and then slice them thinly. Shiitakes are available in many supermarkets, gourmet shops, farmers' markets, health food stores and most Asian food markets.

Reishi mushrooms are not widely available and may have to be ordered by mail. If they come dried, use the same soaking procedure to soften them. If you get canned or fresh reishis, just slice them and add to any recipe calling for mushrooms.

For more information about where to get both types of immunity-boosting mushrooms, contact the Alabama Shiitake Grower's Association, c/o Hosea Hall, Cooperative Extension Service, Alabama A & M University, Box 967, Normal, AL 35762 or Uncle John's Mushroom Company, P.O. Box 491, Doe Run Road, Unionville, PA 19375.

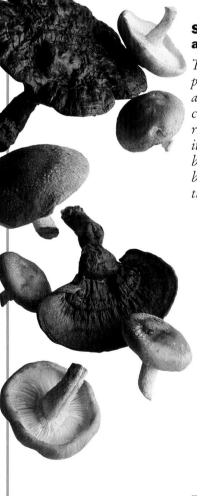

Stir-Fried Shrimp and Mushrooms

This stir-fry is low-fat and easy to prepare, and it may help protect you against infection. You can use any combination of mushrooms in this recipe. But remember, it's the shiitake and reishi varieties that have been shown to contain immunity-boosting compounds. So the more of those you add, the better.

- 6 **tablespoons water**
- 2 **tablespoons low-sodium soy sauce**
- 2 **tablespoons rice wine vinegar**
- 2 **teaspoons honey**
- 2 **teaspoons cornstarch**
- 1 **teaspoon minced garlic**
- 1 **teaspoon minced fresh ginger**
- 1 **teaspoon sesame oil**
- 8 **ounces peeled and deveined medium shrimp**
- 3 **cups small broccoli florets**
- 3 **cups sliced mushrooms (mixed varieties)**
- 1 **cup thinly shredded bok choy leaves**
- 2 **teaspoons toasted sesame seeds**

In a 1-quart saucepan, mix the water, soy sauce, vinegar, honey and cornstarch until the cornstarch has dissolved. Stir in the garlic and ginger. Bring to a boil, stirring constantly, over medium heat. Cook, continuing to stir, for 2 minutes, or until the sauce thickens. Set aside.

Place a wok or large frying pan over medium-high heat until hot. Add the oil.

Swirl the pan to lightly coat the bottom with the oil. Add the shrimp and stir-fry for 2 minutes, or until the shrimp turn pink. Remove the shrimp with a slotted spoon and set aside.

Add the broccoli to the pan and stir-fry for 3 minutes.

Add the mushrooms. Stir-fry for 3 minutes, or until the broccoli is crisp-tender. Add the bok choy; stir-fry for 30 seconds. Add the shrimp and mix well.

Stir in the sauce mixture and mix well to coat the ingredients. Sprinkle with the sesame seeds. Serve immediately.

Makes 4 servings.

Per serving: 203 calories, 3.6 g. fat (15% of calories), 2.4 g. dietary fiber, 87 mg. cholesterol, 443 mg. sodium.

BREAST IS BEST FOR BABY

Breast-feeding may not always be a picnic for new moms, but it offers Junior a smorgasbord of benefits. The first food you can give your child is also one of the best: Various studies show that breast-fed babies have stronger immunity than their formula-fed counterparts. They get less diaper rash and fewer other childhood ailments as well. Researchers from the University of Alberta in Edmonton even found that breast-fed babies respond to disease-protecting immunizations more effectively than children on formula.

Why? Breast milk is richer in some nutrients and contains others in a form that is more easily used by the infant. It is lower in protein and higher in selenium—and it has a form of iron that's superior to the iron in cow's milk. But even when infant formulas match these nutrient amounts, researchers at Pennsylvania State University in University Park found that breast-fed babies still have health advantages. That's because mother's milk also contains a host of hormones, enzymes and other nonnutritional compounds that help boost the production of several antibodies. And those antibodies are important, because they're the guardians that snag bacteria before they can cause infection or disease.

Heightened immunity to several diseases lasts well beyond infancy. There's evidence that breast-feeding may help protect against chronic diseases later in life, including adult-onset diabetes and certain forms of cancer.

Breast-fed babies not only have stronger immunity than their formula-fed counterparts, they even score higher in later years on standardized IQ tests..

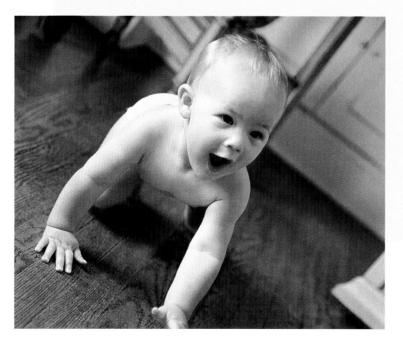

use to make sure you boost your zinc without clogging your arteries? Here are some ways.

Dive into oysters. While various fish and shellfish are rich in zinc, no food comes close to oysters, says Dr. Prasad. A single serving—a half-dozen medium oysters—contains over 75 milligrams of zinc. In fact, just one oyster provides close to your entire daily requirement.

Hoof it over the meat counter—at least occasionally. You may be trying to cut down the amount of meat you eat in order to reduce fat in your diet, but don't cut it out completely. "It's tough for vegetarians to get enough zinc, because some of the best sources are animal proteins," says Dr. Prasad. Beef, lamb and veal are great sources of zinc, with roughly five to seven milligrams in each three-ounce serving.

"In moderation, red meats are fine—even for people trying to reduce the fat in their diets," says Dr. Phillips. But to get the most nutrients with the least fat per bite, choose lean cuts of red meat like beef top round—which has about five milligrams of zinc and four grams of fat per serving. And if you're not into red meat, chicken and turkey are also fine sources of zinc.

Nonmeat sources of zinc include eggs, whole grains, wheat germ, potatoes, pumpkin seeds, green beans and legumes such as lima beans and peas.

Watch your iron intake. Zinc and iron have something of a seesaw relationship, says Dr. Prasad. "Iron and zinc interfere with the absorption of each other. In particular, iron supplements interfere with zinc absorption, making that mineral unavailable to your body." There is no way around this—you need iron for strong immunity. But this can mean trouble for menstruating women, who lose iron during menstrual bleeding. In fact, they may require iron supplements to keep from becoming anemic.

"I guess the best advice is that if you're a woman taking iron supplements, realize you need to eat more

Make Your Own Immunity-Boosting Yogurt

Yogurt has been shown to stop infection where it often begins—in the digestive tract. That's because the live cultures in yogurt contain a substance that activates the immune system to fight infection. You can make your own yogurt with two ingredients—skim milk and live culture powder (available at most health food stores). Just follow the steps shown at right.

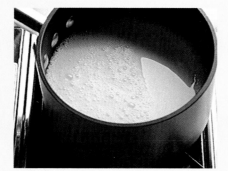

1. Bring one quart of milk to a low boil in a saucepan. When the bubbles are forming, lower the temperature to about 104°F. Test it with a thermometer.

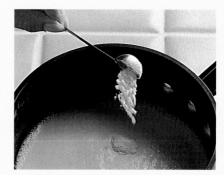

2. Then stir in the powdered yogurt culture.

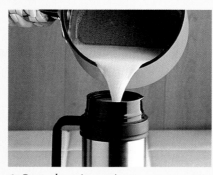

3. Pour the mixture into a vacuum bottle to hold in the heat.

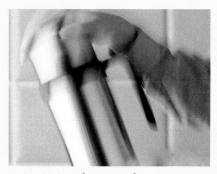

4. Let it sit eight to nine hours or overnight. Before serving, shake the bottle.

DON'T DEPEND ON FROZEN VARIETIES

Some frozen yogurts do contain active bacteria cultures that help boost immunity and fight infection. The bad news is, there's not enough of them to do much good.

"The cultures set up a certain amount of acidity, which makes the characteristic sour flavor," says Manfred Kroger, Ph.D., professor of food sciences at Pennsylvania State University in University Park. So unless your frozen yogurt tastes especially sour—and most don't—you're not getting the same immunity boosters that you get from regular, nonfrozen, tart-tasting yogurt.

foods rich in zinc," says Dr. Prasad. (Men rarely need iron supplements because they usually get enough iron in their diets.)

Go for quality sex, not quantity. Even sex can interfere with levels of zinc in your body. "If you're a man who ejaculates a lot, you're probably zinc deficient," says James Hebert, Sc.D., associate professor of medicine and epidemiology at the University of Massachusetts Medical School in Worcester.

For a reason that's not very well understood, the male reproductive tract concentrates zinc at levels 100 times the concentration found in the blood. For every ejaculation, you lose about one-third the zinc lost from all other sources combined, about 0.63 milligrams each time. This zinc depletion only occurs in the male reproductive tract and doesn't affect women when they reach orgasm.

PROTEIN—AND MORE

The ideal diet for building immunity is the same as a prescription for healthful eating. "Probably the best diet for immunity is the diet we should all be eating, one that's healthful, low in fat and contains all the major nutritional components—proteins, carbohydrates and even a little fat," says Dr. Phillips. "Proteins are important because they help make antibodies and rebuild cells. Carbohydrates are also needed, since they supply the main energy base for all this rebuilding. And fats are essential for being refabricated into the cell membranes; they also are needed for energy.

"But one of the most overlooked—and important—aspects of eating for stronger immunity is to get plenty of the 'micro' nutrients that everybody has to worry about but nobody ever does," he

(continued on page 130)

11 Ways to Sip Away the Sniffles

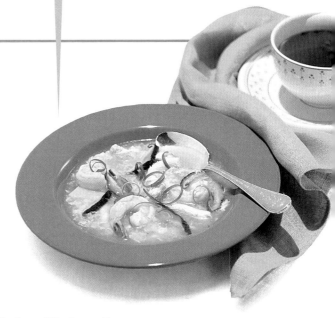

There's plenty of evidence to show that soups, teas and juices can help you get over colds and even flu more quickly—and may even offer some added protection in preventing them. Here's an anti-sniffle smorgasbord.

HOT SOOTHERS— A DIFFERENT CUP O' TEA

Any hot liquid helps cut congestion, says Frederick Ruben, M.D., professor of medicine at the University of Pittsburgh. When you drink something hot, it also raises the temperature in the throat, which slows viral reproduction. But these teas have a bonus: They require no bags and contain no caffeine.

Parsley Tea
Add 2 teaspoons of dried parsley to 1 cup of boiling water. Steep for 10 minutes. You can pour the tea through a strainer to take out the parsley.

Sage Tea
Add 1 teaspoon of dried sage leaves to 1 cup of boiling water. Steep for 10 minutes and pour through a strainer to remove the leaves.

Vinegar 'n' Honey
Mix 1 tablespoon of apple cider vinegar and 1 tablespoon of honey in a cup of hot water.

Hot Lemon Tea
Add 1 or 2 tablespoons of lemon juice to 1 cup of boiling water and stir in honey to taste.

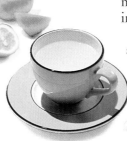

MMMM-MMM, GOOD SOUPS

Breathing vapors from hot soup helps open clogged nasal passages. Then, when you eat the soup, it helps thin mucus to ease congestion and add much-needed nutrients. Mom's chicken noodle soup is still on the cold-curing list, but some other soups are even better—namely those with capsaicin, pepper, mustard and other "hot" ingredients. The hot spices help clear a stuffy nose, while the soothing, nutrient-filled soup gives your virus-fighting ability a boost.

Spicy Shrimp Soup

- 2 cups water
- ½ ounce dried shiitake mushrooms
- 1 boneless, skinless chicken breast half (4 ounces)
- 3 cups defatted chicken stock
- ½ cup bamboo shoots, cut into thin strips
- 2 tablespoons rice wine vinegar
- 2 tablespoons low-sodium soy sauce
- 2 teaspoons grated fresh ginger
- 1 teaspoon sesame oil
- ½ teaspoon ground black pepper
- ¼ teaspoon dry mustard
- ⅛ teaspoon ground red pepper
- 8 ounces peeled and deveined medium shrimp

In a 1-quart saucepan, combine the water and mushrooms. Bring to a boil over high heat. Cover, remove from the heat and set aside to soak.

Meanwhile, place the chicken between two sheets of plastic wrap and flatten to ¼" thickness using a meat mallet or rolling pin. Cut the meat lengthwise into thin strips and crosswise into bite-size pieces.

In a 2-quart saucepan, mix the stock, bamboo shoots, vinegar, soy sauce, ginger, oil, black pepper, mustard and red pepper. Bring to a boil over high heat. Add the chicken and stir to separate the pieces. Reduce the heat to medium-low and simmer for 10 minutes, or until the chicken is cooked through.

Drain the mushrooms, pouring the liquid into the pan with the chicken. Remove and discard any mushroom stems; thinly slice the caps and add them to the pan.

Add the shrimp and cook for 2 minutes, or until the shrimp turn pink and are cooked through.

Makes 4 servings.

Per serving: 154 calories, 3.7 g. fat, (22% of calories), 1 g. dietary fiber, 104 mg. cholesterol, 471 mg. sodium.

Cajun Broth

- 4 cups defatted chicken stock
- 2 bay leaves
- ½ teaspoon dried rosemary, crumbled
- ½ teaspoon dried oregano
- ½ teaspoon dried basil
- ¾ teaspoon paprika
- ¼ teaspoon ground red pepper
- ¼ teaspoon ground black pepper

In a 2-quart saucepan, combine the stock, bay leaves, rosemary, oregano and basil. Bring to a boil over high heat. Reduce the heat to medium-low, cover and simmer for 10 minutes. Stir in the paprika, red pepper and black pepper. Simmer for 5 minutes. Remove and discard the bay leaves.

Makes 4 servings.

Per serving: 19 calories, 0.1 g. fat (5% of calories), 0 g. dietary fiber, 0 mg. cholesterol, 470 mg. sodium.

COLD QUENCHERS

Cool drinks help keep mucous membranes moist and prevent dehydration. Those high in vitamin C and other nutrients also replenish lost vitamins and feed your ailing immune system. Here are some of the best beverages for colds or flu.

Four-Fruit Frenzy

- 2½ cups apple cider
- ¾ cup cranberries
- 1 medium banana, sliced
- ½ cup strawberries
- ¼ cup sunflower seeds

Place the cider, cranberries, bananas, strawberries and sunflower seeds in a blender and process until smooth.

Makes 4 servings.

Per serving: 153 calories, 4.7 g. fat (28% of calories), 1.5 g. dietary fiber, 0 mg. cholesterol, 1 mg. sodium.

Citrus Combo

- 2 cups grapefruit juice
- 2 cups orange juice
- ¼ cup lime juice
- Mint sprigs

In a pitcher, mix all the juices. Serve over ice and garnish with the mint.

Makes 4 servings.

Per serving: 108 calories, 0.4 g. fat (3% of calories), 1.2 g. dietary fiber, 0 mg. cholesterol, 3 mg. sodium.

V-4 Cocktail

- 4 cups tomato juice
- 2 stalks celery, thinly sliced
- 2 tablespoons minced green peppers
- 2 tablespoons lemon juice
- 1 tablespoon minced onions
- 1 teaspoon minced fresh parsley
- ¼ teaspoon crushed celery seeds

Place 1 cup of the tomato juice in a blender. Add the celery, peppers, lemon juice, onions, parsley and celery seeds. Blend until smooth. Stir in the remaining 3 cups tomato juice and chill.

Makes 4 servings.

Per serving: 49 calories, 0.2 g. fat (3% of calories), 3.19 g. dietary fiber, 0 mg. cholesterol, 43 mg. sodium.

Orange Juicy

- 1 can (6 ounces) orange juice concentrate, thawed
- 1 cup water
- 1 cup skim milk
- 2 tablespoons honey
- 1 teaspoon vanilla
- ⅛ teaspoon almond extract
- 4 cups ice cubes

In a blender, combine the orange juice concentrate, water, milk, honey, vanilla and almond extract. Blend on high for 30 seconds. Then gradually drop in the ice cubes and blend until the mixture is smooth.

Makes 4 servings.

Per serving: 138 calories, 0.2 g. fat (1% of calories), 0.3 g. dietary fiber, 1 mg. cholesterol, 35 mg. sodium.

Banana Smoothie

- 2 medium bananas, sliced
- 1 can (8 ounces) crushed pineapple, with juice
- 1 cup crushed ice
- ½ cup orange juice
- 1 container (8 ounces) low-fat vanilla yogurt

In a blender, combine the bananas, pineapple (with juice), ice and orange juice. Blend on high until smooth. Add the yogurt and process until blended.

Makes 4 servings.

Per serving: 134 calories, 1.2 g. fat (7% of calories), 1.6 g. dietary fiber, 3 mg. cholesterol, 40 mg. sodium.

adds. He points out that there are many lesser-known vitamins and minerals that also help nourish the immune system.

Here are some suggestions for getting some of these other much-needed, immunity-boosting nutrients.

Cry fowl. Chicken, turkey, goose and other fowl are great sources of vitamin B$_6$, which is crucial to strong immunity—especially as you age. "When older people were fed diets deficient in B$_6$, their immunity was lowered substantially," says Jeffrey Blumberg, Ph.D., associate director of the U.S. Department of Agriculture (USDA) Human Nutrition Research Center on Aging at Tufts University in Boston. "When their intake was then increased one step at a time, immunity gradually returned to normal." Other good sources of B$_6$ include dark leafy vegetables (also a great source of immunity-building beta-carotene), bananas and prune juice.

Follow the folate. Good sources of folate include dark leafy vegetables, eggs, legumes and salmon. (Liver is another good source, but this organ meat is way too high in fat and cholesterol.) Since folate is needed for overall immunity boosting, you're helping to punch out antigens every time you have a serving of spinach, peas or beans.

Select foods with selenium. That's pretty easy, since this trace mineral is found—if only in the smallest amounts— in virtually every food we eat. Selenium, which like beta-carotene has antioxidant properties, is believed to activate infection-fighting cells and prevent oxidative damage to cells.

"There's been a lot of interest in selenium recently for its possible role in boosting immunity and preventing cancer," says Dr. Garewal of the Arizona Cancer Center. "There was a study in China, where there is a very high rate of gastric cancer. Researchers did a randomized study of 16 vitamins and minerals. They found that groups that received beta-carotene, selenium and vitamin E had a very significant reduction in gastric cancer as well as increased survival."

Whole-grain cereals and breads are good sources—but expect a wide variance in the amount. (That's because selenium is in the soil, and different parts of the country have different amounts.) Selenium is also in animal products such as fish.

Begin your day with milk and magnesium. Most ready-to-eat cereals are fortified with extra nutrients, giving you a lot of what you need for strong immunity—including magnesium, which keeps the immune system from becoming overstimulated and killing healthy cells. A bowl of shredded wheat with skim milk and a banana is an easy way to get over one-third of your daily quota for magnesium. Other good sources of this mineral include leafy vegetables, potatoes, whole grains and seafood.

THE FAT FACTOR

The link may be better established in heart disease, cancer and scores of other illnesses, but research seems to indicate that dietary fat may also worsen an innocent cold or slow healing of wounds.

"There is no question that a low-fat diet is important for strong immunity," says William Adler, M.D., chief of medical immunology at the National Institute on Aging in Bethesda, Maryland.

Various studies by scientists at the USDA Western Human Nutrition Research Center in San Francisco reveal that the more fat in your diet, the less effective your immune system. "All things being equal, the less fat you eat, the stronger your immunity to disease," says Darshan Kelley, Ph.D., research leader of these studies.

Fat may begin to interfere with immunity the moment it's absorbed into cells. "Cells recognize each other by the configuration of proteins on their surfaces," says Dr. Hebert, the first researcher to show the benefits that a low-fat diet has on immunity. "And what fat does, I think, is interfere with the surface so cells can't recognize each other." When the infection-fighting cells aren't

THE RIGHT DIET CAN HELP DELAY AIDS

Eating a diet that's low in fat and high in certain key nutrients may help those infected with HIV to delay the onset of full-blown AIDS, says University of Massachusetts epidemiologist Dr. James Hebert, who first wrote on the link between diet and this deadly disease in 1988.

"The key nutrients appear to be immunity enhancing and have antioxidant properties—namely beta-carotene, ascorbic acid (vitamin C) and vitamin E," says Dr. Hebert.

These nutrients are believed to inhibit the kind of cell activity that allows the virus to spread and eventually shuts down the body's immunity. The most important of these, according to Dr. Hebert, is probably beta-carotene. "This isn't to say that by eating plenty of fruits and vegetables rich in these vitamins, you will avoid AIDS altogether, but you may be able to delay its clinical symptoms," says Dr. Hebert.

able to tell the good guys from the bad guys, researchers speculate, they lose their advantage.

The problem is, many of the foods that help build immunity, like meat, are also high in fat. But here's how to get the nutrition you need for a top-notch immune system without having to go to the last notch on your belt.

Don't try to go too low. There's no need to go overboard in the low-fat department. "Very-low-fat diets don't taste very good, so it's very unlikely that you'll stay on them very long," says Dr. Adler. "My feeling is that if you're able to maintain a fat intake on the lower end of a normal range, then you're not going to feel that you're sacrificing. You'll be able to stay on that eating plan for a long time."

His advice: Try to get between 20 and 30 percent of your total calories from fat sources. This is in contrast to the typical 35 percent or more in the American diet. "This can be accomplished fairly easily, simply by watching your intake of animal sources like fatty meats, ice cream and butter," says Dr. Adler.

Don't butcher up your menu. If you're used to having at least one daily meal that includes meat, there's an easy rule of thumb for building an immunity diet. Try to limit animal sources—even lean ones—to one three-ounce serving two or three times a week.

"Most Americans eat way too much meat, and as a result, they get three to four times as much protein as they need," says Dr. Watson of the University of Arizona College of Medicine.

On the other hand, there's no need to give up meat altogether if you haven't already. "Fish and lean meats like chicken contain a lot of nutrients, so don't feel as though you have to avoid them entirely," says Dr. Adler.

Get productive with produce. "The best way to get the nutrients you need for strong immunity without a lot of fat is to make fresh fruits and vegetables the focus of your diet," says Dr. Hebert. Most produce is nutrient dense,

meaning that it has a lot of vitamins and minerals per bite, with few calories and little fat. There are a few exceptions, such as coconuts, that are high in fat, "but generally, a diet rich in fruits and vegetables will give you what you need for stronger immunity," says Dr. Hebert.

Follow the seasons. One way to keep a fruits-and-veggies diet interesting, says Dr. Adler, is to follow the seasons of freshness: "When you were a kid, your parents might have forced you to eat fruits and vegetables, which is one reason why many people don't like to do it now. But I've found that by following the seasons, you become more educated to freshness, and as a result, enjoy eating produce more. Buy apples in autumn and peaches in summer—whatever is in season. That way, you'll get the best tastes at the best time."

Lose the booze. Alcohol seems to impair the immune system. "Even occasional drinking may displace certain key nutrients—especially the antioxidant and B vitamins," says Dr. Watson. "Moderate or heavy drinking definitely reduces the absorption of these vitamins and suppresses the immune system." That means that you'd have to eat more foods rich in these key nutrients in order to keep your immune system from suffering.

EDIBLE REMEDIES

There's little doubt that the right diet can make you more resistant to disease. But what should you do once a bug has bitten?

Well, it all depends on the ailment. Viruses respond better to food than bacteria, which may require antibiotics. But here's some food for thought—or rather, recovery—the next time these common ailments start ailing you.

Down some C for quicker cold relief. You probably know that vitamin C helps prevent and treat colds. What you may not know, however, is how much extra vitamin C you should add to your diet when you feel a case of the sniffles starting up.

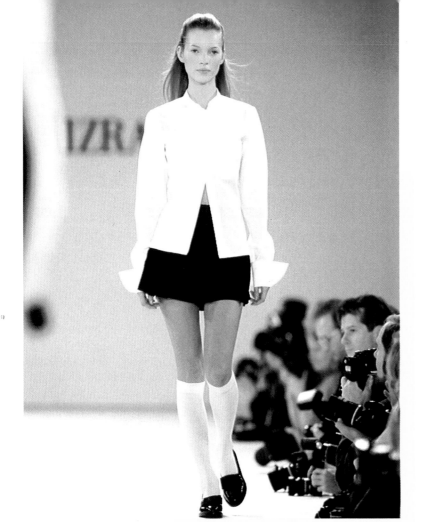

Model behavior? Hardly: Studies show that too-strict dieting— epitomized by many glamorous models of the fashion world—can dampen immunity and leave you vulnerable to disease.

DRASTIC DIETING WEAKENS DEFENSES

Don't let the skinny torsos and cellulite-free thighs of those super-lean models inspire you to take extreme actions: Crash dieting can wreck your immunity. "When you restrict calories severely and suddenly, it depresses immune response," says USDA researcher Dr. Darshan Kelley, one of the nation's foremost authorities on dieting and immunity. "Whenever you go on a diet, you need to ease into it."

The best route? A diet that emphasizes low-fat eating and shoots for a slow but steady weight loss of one to two pounds a week. Liquid diets and other programs that promise faster weight loss can weaken immunity and overall health by depriving you of much-needed food. (Besides, the weight usually comes back.) "I advise that you avoid any diet that's 1,000 calories a day or less," says Dr. Kelley.

The answer: "Studies show it takes about 500 milligrams to reduce sneezes and colds in cold sufferers," says Jeffrey Jahre, M.D., clinical assistant professor of medicine at Temple University School of Medicine in Philadelphia and chief of the Infectious Disease Section at St. Luke's Medical Center in Bethlehem, Pennsylvania. You'll get that amount in about five glasses of a vitamin C–rich juice, such as orange, pineapple, tomato or grapefruit, or in five oranges or large acerola cherries.

Have hot pepper when bronchitis bothers you. Another common virus that strikes nearly everyone at some point is bronchitis, known for producing some of the nastiest-looking phlegm you'll ever see. But eat spicy, and you can help bring an early end to this aggravating ailment.

Foods like hot peppers and curry help thin mucus, making it easier to cough up phlegm, says Varro Tyler, Ph.D., professor of pharmacognosy at Purdue University in West Lafayette, Indiana, who has done extensive research on the use of herbs and traditional remedies.

In fact, spicy foods are good for any kind of congestion, including a stuffy nose. The general rule is, if it will make your eyes water, it will have the same effect *inside* your body.

Use the magic of milk to conquer cold sores. Get the herpes simplex virus and you have a potential problem for life—cold sores (which are also known as fever blisters). These blisters come and go—usually during times of stress or when immunity is low—and usually occur on the outside of your lips. They can also affect your nose, cheeks or fingers.

With an overall healthy diet you may be able to avoid these outbreaks, which usually last a week to ten days. But once they hit, applying whole milk (skim won't work) to the wound can speed recovery. Allow the milk to sit at room temperature before placing a compress directly on the wound, sug-

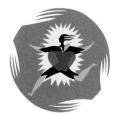

BREAKTHROUGHS IN HEALING

1 8 7 8

Louis Pasteur—along with Jules Joubert and Charles Chamberland—publishes his first paper on *The Germ Theory of Disease,* in which he claims that infectious disease results from germs that invade the body from outside sources such as food or water.

1 9 2 5

One of the earliest food/immunity links is made when Philadelphia researcher C. M. Jackson discovers that malnourished people have an inactive thymus, resulting in a weakened immune system.

1 9 8 9

James Hebert, Sc.D., associate professor of medicine and epidemiology at the University of Massachusetts Medical School in Worcester, discovers that dietary fat seems to depress natural killer cell activity, while a low-fat diet appears to increase resistance to some kinds of infection and disease.

1 9 9 2

Immunity researcher Ranjit Chandra, M.D., of Memorial University of Newfoundland reports that elderly people who supplement certain nutrients in their diets get half the infectious diseases of others who don't supplement these nutrients.

gests Jerome Z. Litt, M.D., assistant professor of dermatology at Case Western Reserve University School of Medicine in Cleveland.

Also limit your intake of foods rich in arginine, an amino acid found in chocolate, cola, peas, cereals, peanuts, gelatin and beer. During outbreaks, avoid these foods altogether, since arginine "feeds" the herpes virus and may trigger cold sores.

Cancel canker sores with yogurt. One of the best ways to avoid these annoying white ulcers with red borders that invade your tongue, gums or the inside of your cheeks is to make yogurt a daily routine.

"Eat at least four tablespoons of unflavored yogurt every day, and you'll prevent canker sores," advises Dr. Litt. It's believed that the beneficial bacteria contained in live-culture yogurt zap canker sores, which seem to strike during times of stress. (If the yogurt contains live cultures, the label will say so.)

Other experts say you may be able to avoid canker sores by eating more foods rich in vitamin C, such as broccoli, cantaloupe and red peppers. Stay away from acidic vitamin C foods like citrus fruits while you have a canker sore, though, because the irritation from the acid will cause you more pain.

Get sweet revenge on yeast infections—avoid sugar. The ever-so-common *Candida albicans* fungus is the culprit behind yeast infections, which can try your immune system as you attempt to relieve that bothersome itch and burning. Yogurt is one way of handling this common form of vaginitis; the active cultures fight the *Candida.* A diet rich in vitamin C is also advised.

But if you're prone to common and stubborn yeast infections, try to put a lid on your sweet tooth. Sugar can cause chronic yeast infections, says Jack Galloway, M.D., clinical professor of obstetrics and gynecology at the University of Southern California School of Medicine in Los Angeles. Brown sugar and honey seem to cause fewer problems than white sugar, but it's still a good idea to limit your intake of candy, cakes and pies.

DON'T GO OVERBOARD

While fish are a good source of immunity-building nutrients, it's possible to get too much of a good thing. Studies show that eating fish every day can weaken the immune system by reducing the ability of some white blood cells to fight infection. Among other immunity problems, daily fish-eaters showed a decrease in the ability of their T-cells to reproduce quickly when faced with an infection.

Lowered immunity may be caused by the very same omega-3 fatty acids that help prevent certain forms of heart disease, say scientists at the U.S. Department of Agriculture Human Nutrition Research Center on Aging at Tufts University in Boston. The researchers believe that adequate levels of antioxidants such as vitamin E and beta-carotene can help reverse the negative effects of the fish oil.

But researchers emphasize that it's only the people who eat fish every day who have problems. "We don't want to discourage people from eating fish," says Tufts nutritional immunologist Dr. Simin Nibbin Meydani, who conducted the test. Instead, she stresses moderation—having fish two or three times a week.

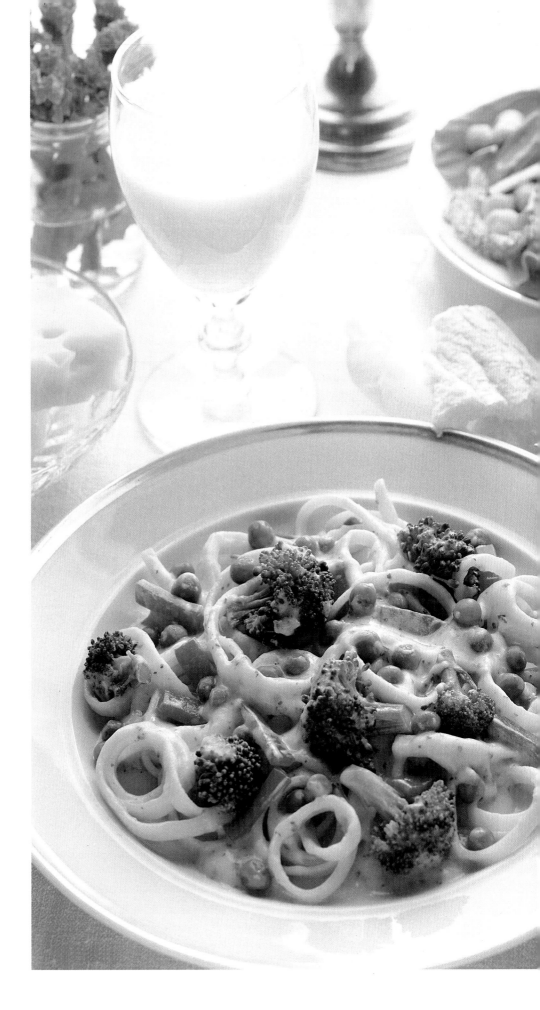

PART FOUR

134

Bone Appetit: Foods for Strength and Pain Relief

Don't

dish it up

unless your

bones can

take it

I f a magician held up a glass of milk and said he could transform it into a knee, a rib or a shoulder, naturally you wouldn't believe him.

If he held up a succulent-looking tenderloin and said this slab of meat could bring searing pain to your fingers, toes and joints, naturally you'd call him a liar.

But the body has some magic methods that simply defy common sense—and it can perform both tricks with the greatest of ease.

The secret of these magic tricks is behind the scenes. In the darkest reaches of the digestive system, the alchemy occurs. And even with years of research, scientists still don't know all the links between food and bone. They know that certain foods may be linked to the pain of arthritis and gout in some people—but why not in others? They know we all have some bone loss as we age—but why do some women have severe osteoporosis while others don't?

Nutritionists would be the first to admit there are some gaps in our knowledge. But on the other hand, a lot of research has paid off in a big way—and doctors can offer authoritative advice on easing joint pain, building stronger bones and avoiding the damage of bone loss. For a taste of their tips—and the advice you need to help ease aching joints and build your body with bone-friendly food—just turn the page.

The Anti-Arthritis Diet

The alarm sounds. Rescue trucks rush to the scene, loaded with special flame-fighting chemicals.

In the first few moments of confusion, it looks like the emergency is well in hand. As the rescue team pours on the fire-dousing chemicals, the fire is reduced to embers.

But what's this? Even while the owner is congratulating the firefighters on a job well done, things start to go wrong with the building. Doors that once opened easily are now stiff and creaky. Windows that once moved up and down smoothly are now groaning. All those exotic chemicals saved the building, only to attack the hinges and joints of the venerable structure.

Time for repairs.

THE BODY'S BOTCHED RESCUE

Like the chemicals that save the building but damage the joints and hinges, your body's immune system sometimes starts a rescue operation that later goes wrong. Cells that fight inflammation rush to the site of the problem—typically a knee or an elbow—but in the process of putting out the fire, they start to whittle away at the cushioning membrane in the joint. Pretty soon there's a new problem—rheumatoid arthritis—causing nasty inflammation and pain in susceptible joints.

Rheumatoid isn't the only kind of

RHEUMATOID ARTHRITIS: WHY JOINTS GET CREAKY

Unlike osteoarthritis, which is caused by wear and tear on joint cartilage, rheumatoid arthritis is caused by an inflammatory reaction. It's triggered by irritation or damage to a joint's synovial membrane, the tissue that lines the joint. The body's immune system rushes enzymes and other substances to heal the damage. But in some people, this process doesn't subside when it should. Tissue is further damaged rather than repaired.

Inflammatory cells and fluids accumulate in the joint, forming a growth called a pannus. This eats into the nearby cartilage, the tough tissue that acts like shock absorbers for our joints. The result is soreness, pain and swelling.

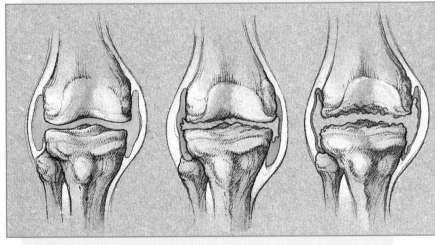

The process begins with the inflammation of the synovial membrane.

A pannus forms, surrounding and eroding nearby cartilage.

In advanced stages, most or all of the cartilage in the joint cavity is destroyed.

arthritis. All in all, there are over 100 types, each dishing out its own brand of misery and discomfort. Some have known causes, while the origins of others remain unknown.

Osteoarthritis is much more common than rheumatoid arthritis, affecting about 60 percent of all arthritis sufferers, or 28 million Americans. Caused by the gradual wearing away of cartilage—the tough material that protects and cushions the bones of a joint—osteoarthritis can cause pain in the joints a number of different ways. For example, pain can result from damage to the bone or damage to the ligaments that hold the bones together.

Gout is a form of arthritis most common among middle-aged men, launching sneak attacks of excruciating pain. The cause is well known: People with gout build up uric acid—a waste product in the blood—and when that crystallizes in a joint, it causes intense inflammation.

At one time, experts believed there was nothing you could do for any of these forms of arthritis except to take some aspirin, rub on a little ice and learn to live with it. But today, rheumatologists (doctors who specialize in treating arthritis and related diseases) are reevaluating the rules of treatment. And for two kinds of arthritis especially—rheumatoid arthritis and gout—doctors have found that a change in diet can often help bring relief.

EATING AROUND THE PROBLEM

Although there is no agreement about a diet to fight rheumatoid arthritis, many researchers say that specific changes in diet can help reduce or prevent arthritis pain in certain people.

"Some people may have a favorable response to a specific diet, but that doesn't mean everyone else will," says Jeffrey R. Lisse, M.D., associate professor of medicine and director of the Division of Rheumatology at the University of Texas Medical Branch in Galveston. "There are a few studies sug-

gesting that some patients with rheumatic diseases may indeed be diet or food sensitive and that this triggers their arthritis flare-ups." But Dr. Lisse emphasizes that there is no single diet that will help large groups of people.

A healthful, balanced diet is the only one that is consistently helpful to most people, he says. He recommends that you talk to your doctor before embarking on any diet plan that calls for the elimination of large groups of foods or that relies heavily on only a few foods.

But while special diets don't provide the answer for most people who suffer from rheumatoid arthritis, other doctors agree that overall good nutrition is definitely a factor in keeping this disease under control.

"There is no doubt that what you eat can modify the function of your immune system," says David Pisetsky, M.D., medical adviser for the Arthritis Foundation and author of *The Duke University Medical Center Book of Arthritis*.

Conversely, poor eating habits can cause the immune system to go on the fritz. Doctors recognize that many allergies, for instance, are related to dietary factors. "Foods are clearly linked to a variety of immune-mediated inflammatory reactions such as asthma, rashes and hives," says Dr. Pisetsky. "It would not be surprising if rheumatoid arthritis, as well as other forms of arthritis, in some people resulted from a similar immune system response."

Dr. Pisetsky recommends that anyone with arthritis should eat a variety of foods and try to maintain ideal weight by eating a low-fat diet. (To find out the maximum amount of fat you should have in your daily diet, see the table on page 44.)

If you do stay at that weight, Dr. Pisetsky points out, your immune system gets all the nutritional benefits it needs. And he says a low-fat weight-loss plan can help stave off bouts of inflammation.

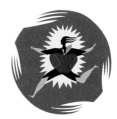

BREAKTHROUGHS IN HEALING

1 9 8 3

Richard S. Panush, M.D., and associates at the University of Florida in Gainesville demonstrate a link between food sensitivity and arthritis. Their findings suggest that arthritis flare-ups and inflammation, in a few people, may be brought on by allergic reactions to certain foods.

1 9 8 5

Joel M. Kremer, M.D., of Albany Medical College in New York, shows that daily intake of omega-3 fatty acids—found in abundance in cold-water fish—reduces the pain and inflammation associated with rheumatoid arthritis.

1 9 9 1

Norwegian researcher Jens Kjeldsen-Kragh, M.D., of the University of Oslo and Norway's National Hospital, demonstrates the effectiveness of fasting followed by a vegetarian diet in reducing rheumatoid arthritis symptoms.

1 9 9 2

The Framingham Knee Osteoarthritis Study concludes that weight loss significantly reduces the risk of osteoarthritis symptoms in women.

DO YOUR KNEES NEED A LIGHTER LOAD?

The majority of those who have osteoarthritis are above their ideal body weight, doctors have found.

"In the course of a day, the human knee is subjected to enormous amounts of stress, which gradually takes its toll on the joint," says Dr. Kenneth Brandt of Indiana University. "Increased weight may increase the stress on the joint. But by losing weight, sometimes even as little as 10 to 15 pounds, stress may be reduced so much that the progression of the disease may be slowed."

Weight control is such an excellent weapon in battling osteoarthritis that doctors frequently encourage people who may benefit from weight loss to drop some extra pounds before considering joint replacement surgery.

GIVING YOUR JOINTS A WEIGHT BREAK

Maintaining ideal weight is especially important for someone who has osteoarthritis, the kind that results from the wearing down of cartilage. Researchers have noted that most cases of osteoarthritis start becoming evident in middle age or later years—which is the same time that most of us begin packing on the pounds. And osteoarthritis is even more likely for those who have been carrying extra weight for longer periods of time—since childhood or young adulthood. Extra body weight places extra stress on your joints.

Joint cartilage eventually breaks down when the stress of moving a load that's too heavy is concentrated in a small area such as the joints, says Kenneth D. Brandt, M.D., professor of medicine and head of the Rheumatology Division at Indiana University School of Medicine in Indianapolis. "Losing just a few pounds can significantly reduce that load and improve the way people feel," he says.

In a long-term Framingham Knee Osteoarthritis study, researchers selected 796 women to study over a ten-year period. The researchers found that those who lost an average of 11 pounds—and kept it off—decreased their risk of developing osteoarthritis by over 50 percent.

In studying groups of obese people (people who are 20 percent over their ideal weight), researchers have shown that weight reduction may reduce pain not only in the knees but also in other joints such as the hips, spine and back. It's also possible that excess weight causes changes in joint cartilage.

And while weight control has been shown to benefit people who have osteoarthritis, it can also help those who have another form of arthritis—gout. Studies show that the likelihood of recurring gout attacks decreases as people lose pounds.

QUENCHING THE FLARE-UPS

In their hunt for foods that cause rheumatoid arthritis, doctors have tried putting people on a limited fast—where calorie intake sometimes went as low as 800 calories a day for a few days or a couple of weeks. Results have been remarkable. Many people with rheumatoid arthritis seem to experience relief when they're fasting.

The trouble is, no one can stay on a fast very long without ending up famished, and what's worse, undernourished. So long-term fasting is not recom-

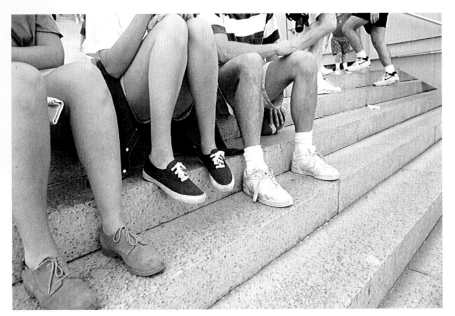

Knees come in all sizes and shapes, but all are vulnerable to the accumulated wear and tear of osteoarthritis.

mended. "Anyone going on an unsupervised, extended fast, even though they may enjoy some benefits in the short term, run the risk of malnutrition that can not only worsen their arthritis in the long run but can put their overall health in jeopardy," says Dr. Pisetsky. He recommends that before you even consider this tactic as a way to stop arthritis, you should definitely review it with your doctor.

The success of fasting raises some interesting questions, however. Is it possible that certain foods aggravate some people's arthritic joints—just as an allergy to certain foods makes some people break into hives or experience shortness of breath? And what if you remove these foods? Will you also reduce the likelihood of recurring rheumatoid symptoms?

Doctors once scoffed at the notion that food allergies could cause flare-ups. But studies have confirmed that some people definitely have allergies that connect with arthritis in some way.

In one landmark study, researchers at the University of Florida in Gainesville tested a woman who claimed that her rheumatoid arthritis acted up whenever she had milk. They filled some food capsules with freeze-dried milk powder and others with nondairy food powder. All the capsules looked the same.

When the woman ate the nondairy food capsules, she had no increase in her arthritis symptoms. When she took the milk-powder capsules, on the other hand, symptoms of morning stiffness, joint swelling and joint tenderness increased, peaking 24 to 48 hours later. In the study, researchers repeated the test four times, and the results were confirmed each time.

Subsequent studies have yielded similar results for some people with allergies to milk as well as other foods. Nevertheless, the percentage of arthritis sufferers who react this way is very small. One expert estimates that only about 5 percent of those with rheumatoid arthritis are food sensitive.

ALLERGIES: NOTHING TO SNEEZE AT

Among the foods that frequently produce reactions in people with rheumatoid arthritis are many that are high in nutrients. So before you drop any food group from your diet, be sure to talk to your doctor to find out whether you'll need supplements to make up for dietary losses.

If you decide to go on an elimination diet—that is, eliminating nearly all foods and then gradually reintroducing food groups one at a time—read "How to Be a Food Detective" on pages 140 and 141 to find out how to do it. Here are some actions you might want to take if you think your problems are associated with some of the foods you commonly eat.

Nix the tomato. In a dietary study conducted by researchers in Israel, tomatoes caused symptoms in 22 percent of the patients suffering from rheumatoid arthritis. If you find you have to avoid this vegetable, you'll also have to stay away from ketchup, tomato sauce and other products that contain tomatoes. Also be sure to check labels on soups and prepared foods.

Give the red light to red meat. People who are allergic to red meat may need to avoid all kinds—pork, lamb and game meats as well as beef. This may seem like a loss at first, until you get used to a vegetarian diet. If you do find that red meat is part of the problem, be sure to look at the plan for switching to a vegetarian diet on pages 144 to 147.

Deny the dairy. In the dietary study in Israel, researchers also found that milk caused symptoms in 37 percent of rheumatoid arthritis patients, and cheese affected 24 percent. As this study demonstrated, dairy products such as milk, cheese and butter can definitely cause flare-ups of rheumatoid arthritis in some people. If dairy foods aggravate your arthritis, read food labels to make sure dairy products are not used in any prepared foods you're eating.

Keep corn and other grains in the outfield. Corn, wheat, oats and rye ag-

How to Be a Food Detective

Are your rheumatoid arthritis flare-ups caused by a hypersensitivity to certain foods? A growing body of evidence suggests that many common foods actually contain allergens, substances that trigger allergic reactions that worsen the severity of arthritis symptoms such as inflammation and stiffness. But which foods contain the allergens that are causing your problems?

To find out, the usual approach is to go on an elimination diet, a doctor-supervised program in which you're put on a total or near-total fast for several days. Ordinary foods are then added back to the diet, one at a time, to determine which ones make your arthritis worse. If symptoms arise following the reintroduction of a specific food, you've nabbed the culprit.

Even after you've started an elimination diet, however, it can take weeks to identify the aggravating food. Also, arthritis symptoms are sometimes slow to develop after a food is reintroduced. And of course, you can't eliminate all foods at the beginning of the diet, or you'd run the risk of malnutrition.

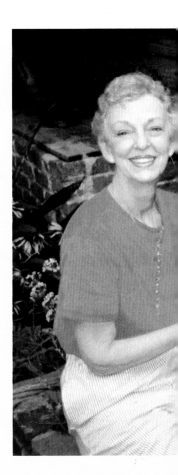

You shouldn't try any drastic dietary manipulations without consulting a physician, advises Dr. David Pisetsky, medical advisor for the Arthritis Foundation. But you can try a safe, modified version of the elimination diet to deduce if something in your diet is triggering your arthritis flare-ups. The following are well-considered steps that doctors recommend.

Keep a diary. It's important to record your body's signals, says Dr. Pisetsky. He suggests that you write down everything you eat. After you've done this a few times, you'll be able to compare lists and see what might have led to flare-ups. Start a list of likely suspects.

Test your hunch. When you've established that a certain food looks like a prime suspect, stop eating it for about a week to get it out of your system. If you feel better, you know you're getting warm. Then try the food again and see if your symptoms worsen. Repeat this test twice: If your symptoms get worse each time, you can be sure you've made a connection.

Think before you banish. If you've identified the aggravating food as something you don't eat

often, you can probably avoid eating it and never know the difference. But if it's a very common or essential part of a balanced diet, such as a dairy product, a meat, a grain or a fruit or vegetable, see a doctor or nutritionist before you quit cold turkey. Don't give up a food unless you're sure another source will give you the nutrients provided by that food.

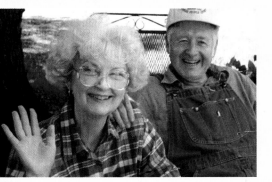

"If I stay away from sugar, I have a lot less pain," says Ruby Nelson of Mahtomedi, Minnesota.

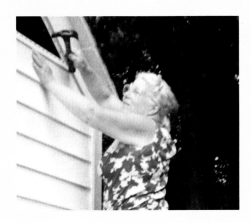

Lahoma Davis of Warren, Texas, discovered that eating red meat made her hands start to swell almost immediately.

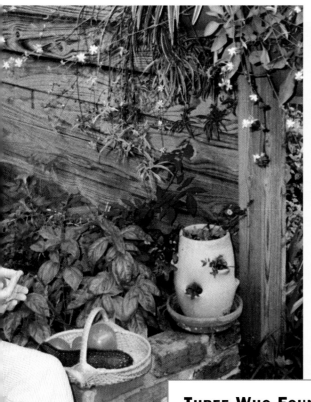

Julia Smith, a gardener from Huntsville, Alabama, found that her fingers would swell whenever she had a helping of tomatoes.

THREE WHO FOUND RELIEF

We talked to several people who had long suspected that food aggravated their arthritis symptoms. With a little homespun detective work, all three were able to pinpoint the culinary culprits.

Lahoma Davis of Warren, Texas, discovered that she was particularly sensitive to red meat, dairy products, sugar and food preservatives. "I am so sensitive that if I eat red meat, my hands start to swell up within ten minutes or so," she says.

Julia Smith, a Huntsville, Alabama, gardener, claims that she grows the best tomatoes around, but she found that her fingers would swell up whenever she ate a bumper crop. "I eat them anyway," she says. "I don't mind a little discomfort."

Ruby Nelson of Mahtomedi, Minnesota, noted a connection with refined sugar. "I don't usually eat sugar, but I noticed that after weekends when we'd had company, and I'd eaten sugar, my knees would swell up for days."

gravate rheumatoid arthritis in some people. Avoiding them is difficult because they're in so many foods—and you'll be missing out on fiber and important nutrients if you try a grain-free menu. But if they're causing the inflammation problem, you may be able to avoid them and—with a doctor's guidance—fill out your menu with other high-fiber foods and supplements to make up for the fiber and nutrients you might be missing.

Line up other suspects. A wide variety of foods has been reported to aggravate rheumatoid arthritis in some people. Citrus fruits such as oranges, grapefruit and lemons occasionally cause problems. And certain people have found that they can't eat eggs without experiencing a flare-up. Others find they have to avoid refined sugar. And a few people are wary of specific foods such as peanuts or certain beverages such as coffee. One way to find out if you're allergic to any one of these foods is to drop it from your menu for a few weeks—and then see what happens.

CHOOSING YOUR FATS WITH CARE

For anyone with rheumatoid arthritis, eating fat-filled foods may lead to painful consequences. Animal fats in meats, dairy products and shellfish produce hormonelike substances called prostaglandins, which are highly inflammatory.

"People can experience dramatic improvements in their symptoms when they cut back on their consumption of high-fat foods such as dairy products and red meats," says the Arthritis Foundation's Dr. Pisetsky.

Across-the-board fat reduction, combined with exercise, can significantly reduce rheumatoid arthritis symptoms, according to a study conducted by Edward H. Krick, M.D., of Loma Linda University in California. Dr. Krick selected 46 people who suffered from rheumatoid arthritis and then placed half the group on a program of exercise and stress reduction. The other half was on the same

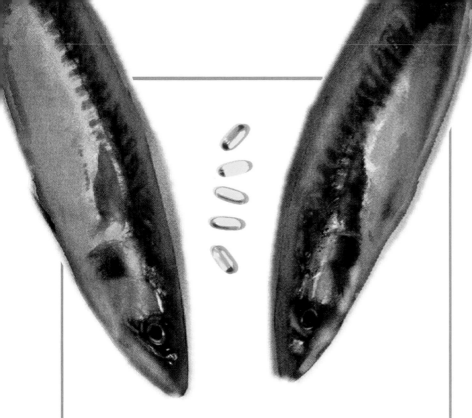

Streamline your intake of omega-3 fatty acids: The amount of oil contained in these five capsules is the equivalent of what you'd get from eating two whole mackerel.

THE EASIER WAY TO TAKE FISH OIL

Many studies have shown that a diet high in omega-3 fatty acids can significantly reduce the inflammation and stiffness associated with rheumatoid arthritis. In most of these studies, participants consumed fish oil containing about three to five grams of omega-3's per day, the equivalent of 8 to 13 ounces of mackerel. Fortunately, there's another way to get your omega-3's: Just take fish-oil capsules, which are available over the counter at almost any pharmacy.

That's good news, but doctors are quick to point out that fish-oil supplements are not a total substitute for the real McCoy. Fish is a low-fat, nutrient-rich food source that should be a staple of most arthritis patients' diets, says Dr. Joel Kremer of Albany Medical College. And frequent use of fish-oil capsules can cause gas.

program plus a very-low-fat diet (10 percent of total calories). After 12 weeks, the low-fat group was significantly better off than the high-fat group in regard to the number of tender and swollen joints.

You probably won't be able to reduce the fat in your daily diet to 10 percent of calories, because that percentage of fat is extremely low. On the other hand, any reduction can help. And of course,

when you eat low-fat, you'll get the benefits of weight loss.

But there is one type of fat that you don't want to cut from your diet—the omega-3 fatty acids found in abundance in the oil of cold-water fish. Omega-3's are thought to work on rheumatoid arthritis by reducing the body's production of inflammatory substances, according to Joel M. Kremer, M.D., professor of medicine and head of the Division of Rheumatology at Albany Medical College in New York. His research has shown that a diet high in omega-3 fatty acids can bring a modest reduction in inflammation.

In one 24-week study of 49 people with rheumatoid arthritis, Dr. Kremer found that those who received high doses of fish oil had significantly less tenderness than those who didn't have any fish oil.

According to Dr. Kremer, physicians have known for years that Eskimos, Scandinavians and other people who get a lot of fish oil in their diets have the lowest rate of rheumatoid arthritis in the world. But that's not the only reason he and other rheumatologists are fish advocates. "I recommend to all my patients that they eat more fish, not just because fish oil is a good anti-inflammatory agent but because it's good for your overall health, too," he says.

Eight to ten ounces of sardines, salmon or tuna contain about the same levels of omega-3 fatty acids used in Dr. Kremer's studies. Other fish high in omega-3's are mackerel, herring, whitefish, anchovies and bluefish.

A PLAN TO KNOCK OUT GOUT

Gout used to be considered an ailment of the rich. Back in the days when royalty ate roast boar while peasants dined on bread and potatoes, gout was the curse of the upper class.

Now we know why. First of all, obesity makes people more susceptible to gout. Also, their diets were high in the compounds known as purines—chemicals that the body converts to uric acid, which is the substance that causes gout attacks.

Today all of us have access to purine-rich foods. "Usually these foods won't cause a gout attack by themselves," observes Christopher M. Wise, M.D., associate professor of internal medicine in the Division of Rheumatology at Virginia Commonwealth University Medical College of Virginia in Richmond. He says certain people are "genetically predisposed" to get arthritis—that is, they have an inherited gene that makes them more vulnerable to purines than others.

"But if you carry that gene, and your diet is very high in purine-rich foods, that could be enough to raise your body's uric acid levels to trigger a gout attack," says Dr. Wise. "And if you continue eating those foods, the likelihood of future attacks will be very high."

Although drugs can keep gout under control, doctors say that even medication is more effective if gout-prone people watch their diets. Here are the strategies.

Pass on purines. Purines are found in many different types of foods, but most have insignificant amounts. You can avoid the worst offenders, including organ meats such as liver and kidneys and foods that contain gravies and meat extracts. Unfortunately, some fish that are very healthful in other respects—including high omega-3 sources such as anchovies, herring and mackerel—also contain purines. It's also wise to avoid high-purine shellfish such as shrimp, scallops, crab, lobster and oysters.

Some vegetables have purines, though not as much as the worst offenders. The ones to watch out for include spinach, asparagus and mushrooms. People with gout should also steer clear of peas, kidney beans, lentils and lima beans.

Gulp those glasses. Dr. Pisetsky recommends that you keep sipping water and other beverages throughout the day. The extra fluid helps flush uric acid out of the body before it can crystallize.

Lose weight, but don't crash-diet. If you're overweight and gout-prone, you should back off on high-fat foods. But the goal is to lose weight gradually. Most doctors advise against going on a starvation-type diet that produces very rapid weight loss.

In fact, a crash diet can aggravate gout rather than help it. "Sudden, rapid burning of body fat can produce high uric acid levels in some people," says Dr. Wise.

Tend toward teetotaling. Gout sufferers should drink alcohol in very small amounts, if at all, says Dr. Wise. That's because alcohol tends to make uric acid levels rise. Another reason: beverages like wine and beer have a high purine content.

GOING TOE TO TOE WITH GOUT

A gout attack occurs when crystals of uric acid, a natural body chemical that is normally excreted, find their way into a joint. Uric acid is a waste product, and if the kidneys can't remove it all, crystals start to form. The crystals settle to the feet and hands like sugar in a teacup.

Sixty percent of initial gout attacks occur in the big toe. But besides attacking the toe, gout can spread to and inflame other joints as well. Some common attack sites include (in order of frequency) the insteps, ankles, heels, knees, wrists, fingers and elbows.

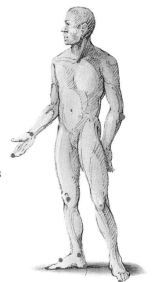

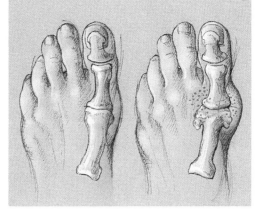

Uric acid crystals are sharp and intensely inflammatory. The accumulation of crystals, called tophi, can be extraordinarily painful.

The Benefits of Meatless Eating

Physicians have long known that fasting is an effective short-term treatment for rheumatoid arthritis. But naturally, you can't fast forever. And unfortunately, most people tend to experience a relapse when the pain-causing food is reintroduced.

But many rheumatologists and researchers recommend a vegetarian diet. They've found that some people who switch to a vegetarian diet can sustain the benefits that come from fasting, even though they start eating again. The difference is, they don't eat everything—just certain vegetarian-type foods.

To see if people on a vegetarian diet would be as pain-free as those who fasted, researchers from the University of Oslo and the National Hospital in Oslo, Norway, set up an experiment involving 53 people, all of whom had arthritis. Dividing the participants into two groups, researchers placed one group on a fast and allowed the other group to eat its usual diet.

During an initial seven- to ten-day fast, participants consumed only herbal teas, garlic, vegetable broth, water and various vegetable juices. After that, researchers gradually introduced the components of a vegetarian diet: noncitrus fruits, vegetables, gluten-free whole grains and legumes. But the participants continued to abstain from any foods that contained meat, fish, eggs, dairy products, gluten (a component found in wheat), refined sugar, salt, spices, preservatives and citrus fruits.

One month from the beginning of the study, people who had started by fasting and then switched to a vegetarian diet reported significant reductions in their arthritis symptoms. They had a decrease in the number of tender joints, less morning stiffness and pain and considerably more grip strength.

After three to five months, the experimental group was allowed to gradually begin eating foods containing gluten, such as breads and wheat products, along with milk and other dairy products. The participants maintained this diet for another eight to ten months.

Finally, after a total of 13 months, researchers compared the group that was now on a full vegetarian diet with the group that had not changed its diet at all. The conclusions were decisive. The symptoms of the group that had stuck to an "ordinary diet" either stayed the same or got worse. But the experimental group reported continued improvement in their symptoms even

On a vegetarian menu, you'll find plenty of foods to please the palate. Shown below is a selection of foods for breakfast, lunch and dinner. (See page 147 for a full menu.)

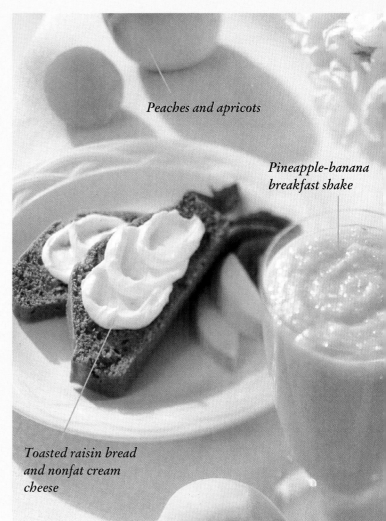

Peaches and apricots

Pineapple-banana breakfast shake

Toasted raisin bread and nonfat cream cheese

when they switched over to a vegetarian diet.

In other words, the benefits of fasting persisted as long as those people continued with their individualized vegetarian diets.

Although a vegetarian diet might not be for everyone, this study shows that it might make a dramatic difference for some people who have very painful symptoms. And if you decide to try fasting, be sure to do it only with a doctor's supervision, particularly if you have other health problems besides arthritis.

VEGGIE PLUSES

Why does a vegetarian diet sometimes take the fire out of inflammation?

Researchers have a few theories. For one thing, people tend to be allergic to fewer substances in vegetables than in meat and dairy products.

Vegetables may also provide benefits because of what they don't contain. "A vegetarian diet is usually low in calories and fat," says Dr. David Pisetsky, medical advisor for the Arthritis Foundation. "We don't know why, but a low-calorie, low-fat diet seems to somehow improve the function of the immune system in some people, and that results in less inflammation and other symptoms."

But if you were brought up to be a true-blue, meat-loving American, the mere mention of the word *vegetarian* may be enough to make you swerve toward the nearest fast-food burger

Grapes

Baked apple with caramel sauce

Romaine salad with chick-peas and low-fat Thousand Island dressing

Cold rice salad with pimiento and pine nuts

Vermicelli with chunky vegetables and Monterey Jack cheese

Split pea soup with toasted croutons

palace. After all, vegetarianism means giving up all the good things in life in favor of twigs, acorns and rabbit food, right?

Wrong.

For most people, making the transition from omnivore to herbivore doesn't really require a major lifestyle adjustment. Today you can go meatless and still enjoy meals that are flavorful, filling and satisfying.

First off, most vegetarian meal plans already consist of foods that you love to eat, such as salads, pasta, potatoes, fresh fruits, breads and corn. So if you think you're going to sacrifice all your favorite foods, you're sorely mistaken.

Besides, vegetarianism doesn't necessarily have to be an all-or-nothing affair. "Most arthritis patients probably don't need to become complete vegetarians to enjoy the benefits that vegetarianism often provides," says Dr. Pisetsky. "Many people benefit simply by incorporating elements of vegetarianism. They cut back somewhat on their red meat or dairy consumption while increasing their fruits and vegetables. Or, if they're sensitive to red meat, they replace it with poultry and fish."

MAKING UP FOR MEAT

If you switch to a vegetarian diet, you might be concerned about getting all of the nutrients you need. But you don't have to worry as long as you get plenty of variety—and include milk and eggs (if you're not allergic to them) as well as vegetables in your diet. Load your diet with vegetarian fare, and you'll meet most of the general nutritional guidelines that everyone—whether they have arthritis or not—should be following to maximize their health, says Dr. Pisetsky.

Plus, there are a number of extra benefits. A vegetarian diet is low in cholesterol. And it's rich in fiber and complex carbohydrates.

It's the strict vegetarian diets—the kinds that allow no fish, dairy products or eggs—that need to be carefully supervised to make sure you get all the nutrients you need.

"When you eliminate meats and dairy products, you eliminate the best sources of certain nutrients," says Dr. Jeffrey Lisse of the University of Texas Medical Branch in Galveston.

But with some planning, you can make up all or most of the nutrients that are found in meats. Here are some guidelines to keep in mind.

■ If you omit all animal products from your diet, you may lack protein. So make sure your diet focuses on protein-rich plant foods such as legumes (beans and peas) and nuts.

■ If you give up meat, you're also giving up the iron, zinc and vitamins that meat provides. You can get more of these vital nutrients by eating legumes, tofu, whole grains, prunes, raisins, spinach, nuts and seeds. Eating fortified cereals and green leafy vegetables will also help give you the vitamins and minerals found in meat.

■ Anyone who cuts out dairy products is giving up the richest source of calcium, which can increase your risk of osteoporosis as well as contribute to further joint damage. You can get a calcium boost from dark green leafy vegetables, tofu, legumes and orange juice fortified with calcium. But depending on your need for calcium, you may also want to take supplements.

■ Vitamin B_{12}, an essential nutrient, is found exclusively in animal foods. If you eliminate eggs, dairy products and meats, you'll have to rely on fortified cereals or supplements to get your daily dose. But if you give up only meat—and not eggs or dairy foods—you'll be more likely to get the B_{12} you need.

A SEVEN-DAY VEGETARIAN MENU

When you plan your meals, you may think of the meat first. And after you've settled on the entrée, you think about the extras that go with it. You take a portion of beef, chicken, lamb or some other meat, then decide what vegetables, soup, salad and bread would be complementary.

Things aren't so clear-cut when you remove the meat from a meal. You may not be sure which foods go together or what dishes will give you enough protein to carry you through the day.

To help you get started, here's an example of a meatless meal plan that's tasty, easy to prepare and rich in all the nutrients your body needs. While this plan is just for one week, it's easy to see how foods can be mixed and varied for a total meal plan that could help ease your arthritis.

DAY	BREAKFAST	LUNCH	DINNER	SNACK
1	Grapefruit sections Raisin bran cereal with low-fat or skim milk	Cheese ravioli with marinara sauce and Parmesan Tossed green salad with chick-peas, carrots and light dressing Fresh fruit salad	Minestrone soup Steamed snow peas Boston lettuce salad with blue cheese dressing Whole-wheat roll Almond cookies	Rice cakes All-fruit preserves
2	Pineapple-banana shake Toasted raisin bread Nonfat cream cheese	Split pea soup with toasted croutons Cold rice salad with pimiento and pine nuts Grapes	Penne pasta with steamed vegetables, chopped olives and mozzarella Grilled eggplant slices Romaine salad with chick-peas and low-fat Thousand Island dressing Baked apple with caramel sauce	Hot chocolate made with low-fat milk
3	Orange juice Apple pancakes with maple syrup	Macaroni and cheese with chopped tomatoes and zucchini Bitter greens with tangy dressing Melon balls	Grilled vegetable patties with lettuce and sliced tomatoes on a whole-wheat bun Baked navy beans Cinnamon graham crackers Skim milk	Raisins and lightly smoked almonds
4	Strawberries Oatmeal	Noodle soup Melba toast Low-fat Monterey Jack cheese Nonfat chocolate pudding	Vermicelli with chunky vegetables Escarole and red onion salad with balsamic vinegar Italian bread rubbed with garlic and drizzled with olive oil Steamed asparagus Sliced kiwi fruit and oranges drizzled with honey	Popcorn
5	Peach nectar Scrambled egg substitute with peppers and onions	Pita stuffed with nonfat cream cheese, shredded carrots and chives Hot couscous with lentils, tomatoes and Parmesan Celery sticks Nonfat pineapple yogurt Apple juice	Vegetable lasagna Steamed snow peas Raw spinach with low-fat Oriental soy dressing Pears	Low-fat Swiss cheese and oat crackers
6	Cranberry juice Vidalia onion omelet Toasted bagel Nonfat cream cheese	Baked potato Hearty lentil chili Mixed green salad with low-fat Dijon dressing Mixed dried fruit	Baked winter squash stuffed with sesame seeds Steamed green beans Tossed green salad with low-fat Oriental soy dressing Raspberry fruit-and-yogurt bar	Dried apple rings
7	French toast Low-fat milk Blueberries	Cheese pizza Roasted red peppers and blanched green beans with balsamic vinegar Nonfat yogurt with raisins, cinnamon and honey	Vegetable kabobs Baked sweet potato Couscous with grated orange peel Banana fruit shake	Ice milk with chopped nuts and pineapple topping

Osteoporosis: Stop Bone Loss Now

I f the human skeleton had just been invented, it would be plugged as the greatest innovation since plastics. Imagine the advertising: "Light! Durable! Lasts for decades!" The superlatives: "Hundreds of flexible joints! Provides years and years of reliable service! Supports 100–200–300 pounds... or even more!" The miraculous claims: "Self-mending! Renewable parts! Totally

BONE DENSITY BASICS

Magnified under the lens of a microscope, a cross-section of bone is honeycombed with thin struts that look like partitions. Threading their way through this honeycomb, bone cells called osteoclasts are constantly dissolving old bone and carrying it out in the bloodstream. Meanwhile, bone cells called osteoblasts fill in these holes with spongy fibers of protein called collagen, which combines with calcium to form crystals. And it's these crystals that make the bone hard. If the doctor says you have "good bone density," it means your bones are thick-walled and closely webbed with struts.

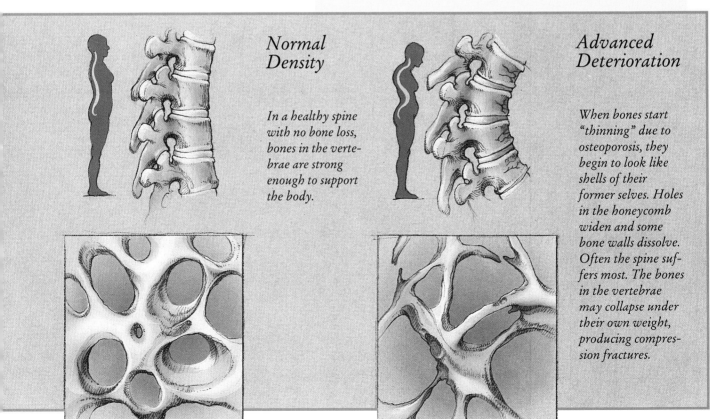

Normal Density

In a healthy spine with no bone loss, bones in the vertebrae are strong enough to support the body.

Advanced Deterioration

When bones start "thinning" due to osteoporosis, they begin to look like shells of their former selves. Holes in the honeycomb widen and some bone walls dissolve. Often the spine suffers most. The bones in the vertebrae may collapse under their own weight, producing compression fractures.

organic! Never needs cleaning!"

A wonderful invention indeed—but then you get to the fine print. Way down in the corner, in very tiny type, you see the caution: "Warning: Certain nutrients are absolutely essential for life-long maintenance of a well-working skeleton. Some groups of people, particularly older women, may have skeletons that are prone to breakage. Whatever your age, be sure to monitor your diet for adequate nutrients."

And then the clincher: "The main danger—which can be partially avoided by good nutrition—is the risk of osteoporosis."

MAINTENANCE TIPS FOR EVERYONE

Osteoporosis is a medical term that comes from the Latin word for "porous bones." Osteoporosis is not something that happens all of a sudden. Instead, it's a long-term process that usually accelerates as we get older.

Doctors know that it's much more likely to affect some people than others, so they can tell you whether you're more at risk than someone of another sex, age or race. To summarize the risk factors: Women get osteoporosis much more frequently than men, and small-framed white women are more susceptible than women of other races and other body types. But doctors also admit that they don't know why.

Some bone thinning is a natural part of aging. Our bodies run less efficiently as we get older, and as the years pass, we don't absorb the nutrients from our food as well as we used to. With osteoporosis the bone-thinning process speeds up as the birthdays fly by. To understand why—and to find out what can slow down that process—doctors have put bone building under the microscope of extensive research. And here's what they've found.

Our bones' chief fodder is calcium. But even though bones are a collection agency for calcium, the body needs calcium for all sorts of work besides building bone. The heart, for example,

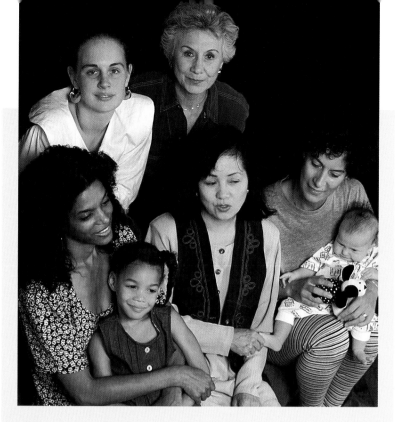

RISK AT A GLANCE

Some of the women shown above have a higher risk of osteoporosis than others. But which ones? Listed below are some of the risk factors that researchers have discovered by studying the incidence of osteoporosis among different populations and age groups.

- You're more at risk if you are Caucasian or Asian.
- Small-framed women are more likely to get osteoporosis than large-framed women.
- Your risk rises when you're over 40, especially during and after menopause.
- Women with children are somewhat less likely to have osteoporosis than women with no children.

For women who are in a high-risk group, it's particularly important to have a bone-density measurement test.

needs calcium to help regulate its beat, and blood needs calcium to assist with clotting. So the skeleton works two jobs: It supports the body, and at the same time it's a storage facility for all the calcium the body uses for dozens of everyday life-functions.

If we don't get enough calcium from our diet—if we flat-out avoid milk and milk products, for example—calcium moves from our bones into our blood.

"The calcium in our bodies is very tightly controlled and regulated in order to maintain that precise level of calcium in the blood," explains Robert Lindsay,

M.D., professor of clinical medicine at the College of Physicians and Surgeons at Columbia University in New York and president of the National Osteoporosis Foundation in Washington D.C. When it comes to calcium, blood has first dibs over bone.

But you don't have to play Solomon and force your body to choose. Proper diet, exercise and calcium supplements can help you prevent at least some of the bone loss.

UNFAIR SELECTION

In the risk polls for osteoporosis, there's no question that women are in the losing party. Osteoporosis creeps up on 45 percent of all Caucasian or Asian women in the United States who are 50 years or older. Men get osteoporosis, too, but not as often—and the bone loss problem shows up about ten years later than it does in women.

Until about age 35 both men and women build more bone than they lose—if they have enough calcium in their diets. Density increases to a maximum called peak bone mass. After age 35, breakdown usually begins, and we slowly lose bone, perhaps as much as 1 percent a year. The goal then is to slow the loss to a bare minimum.

For women, menopause begins a unique danger zone for rapid bone loss—as much as 7 percent a year—for roughly five years. It's caused by declining levels of estrogen, which protects bone density in ways not yet fully understood. Depending on a woman's bone mass entering menopause, this is often the critical period when she crosses the line from strong bones to osteoporotic bones—bones that can fracture under only minor stress. For this reason women always need adequate calcium in their diets—plus supplements, if necessary.

A man is more likely to be 60 than 50 when bone loss accelerates, according to Kenneth H. Cooper, M.D., president and founder of the Cooper Aerobics Center in Dallas and author of *Preventing Osteoporosis*. Among men who are over 75, about one-third have symptoms of osteoporosis.

Adding up all the probabilities, four women develop osteoporosis for every one man. Being at risk doesn't mean you'll necessarily have osteoporosis. But doctors recommend that women in high-risk groups pay special attention to diet, exercise and supplements.

It's also important for women to have a bone-density measurement taken around the time they begin menopause, if not sooner. "If a woman is approaching menopause—say 45 years or more—regardless of her risk factors, there's value to taking stock of her bones at that time in her life," says endocrinologist John Bilezikian, M.D., director of the Metabolic Bone Diseases Program at Columbia–Presbyterian Medical Center in New York. "Whether her bone density is normal, somewhat reduced or markedly reduced can be very important information," he adds. Your physician can refer you to a facility that performs bone-density measurement. And Dr. Bilezikian recommends another test about one year after

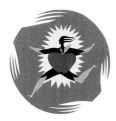

BREAKTHROUGHS IN HEALING

1 9 7 5

Early clinical trials show that calcium supplements of at least 750 milligrams per day slow bone loss in postmenopausal women. Four out of six trials between 1975 and 1981 confirm these findings.

1 9 9 2

Researchers from Indiana University School of Medicine and the Regenstrief Institute for Health Care, both in Indianapolis, study bone loss in 45 pairs of identical twins. The study proves that heredity does not mean you'll automatically get osteoporosis. You can increase bone strength just by getting more calcium in your diet.

1 9 9 3

In Sydney, Australia, a team of scientists discovers the inherited factor that turns on the bone-making process. Scientists believe this discovery will lead to a blood test for osteoporosis. Those at risk can then take earlier preventive measures, increasing calcium and vitamin D in their diets.

the start of menopause to check for the rate of bone loss.

"Bone-density measurement is a better predictor for risk of fracture than either blood pressure is for stroke or cholesterol is for heart disease," says Dr. Lindsay. And if the measurement shows you're at risk, you should talk to your doctor about increasing dietary calcium and taking supplements.

During the first five years after menopause, doctors have found, the most effective weapon against rapid bone loss at this time is hormone-replacement therapy, or HRT—usually a combination of the hormones estrogen and progestin. If the doctor determines that your bone density is "borderline" at the start of menopause, then calcium and exercise are no longer enough by themselves to keep your bones from losing ground. According to Dr. Lindsay, women whose bone density is already low at the onset of menopause should consider using HRT to prevent their existing osteoporosis from becoming more severe.

WHEN THE BONE BREAKS

Osteoporosis robs aging bones with such stealth that it's often called the silent crippler.

"You don't feel your bones becoming weak and fragile," says Laurie Gibson Lindberg, director of patient education and information at the National Osteoporosis Foundation. In fact, the first news that you have osteoporosis may come one morning when you're performing a simple task and something snaps.

An elderly person with osteoporosis—or a younger person who has very advanced osteoporosis—can break a rib just from bending over, according to Clifford R. Rosen, M.D., director of the Maine Center for Osteoporosis Research and Education in Bangor.

Researchers estimate the number of osteoporosis-related fractures at 1.5 million a year. The toughest break is the hip fracture. An older person can end

HOW MUCH IS ENOUGH?

Both the National Osteoporosis Foundation and the National Institutes of Health would like to see Americans—especially women—get more than the Recommended Dietary Allowance (RDA) for calcium. The chart below shows the RDA for various groups of people—and also the higher, ideal levels that are recommended by the National Osteoporosis Foundation.

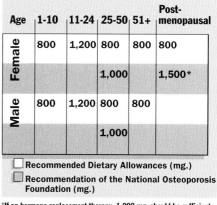

Age	1-10	11-24	25-50	51+	Post-menopausal
Female	800	1,200	800	800	800
			1,000		1,500*
Male	800	1,200	800	800	
			1,000		

☐ **Recommended Dietary Allowances (mg.)**
☐ **Recommendation of the National Osteoporosis Foundation (mg.)**

*If on hormone replacement therapy, 1,000 mg. should be sufficient.

up bedridden after breaking one of the crucial bones in the hip, and that often leads to numerous other complications.

But although 300,000 osteoporosis-related hip fractures occur every year, they are not a natural part of old age. Neither are spine fractures or broken wrists—the other osteoporosis hot spots.

In order to build up bone reserves to see you through later years, it's best to begin early. Calcium, along with vitamin D to help absorption, are critical dietary elements in bone building—and should be accompanied by weight-bearing exercise like walking or low-impact aerobics. Studies show that active children and young men and women who get plenty of calcium in their diet stay above the "fracture threshold." "That means their bone density is so high that, although it will decline, they won't have problems till they're 90—or maybe never," says Dr. Cooper.

(continued on page 154)

Shortcuts to More Calcium

Can we really get all the good-to-the-bone calcium we need from our diet? Right now, only 25 percent of the women in America get the minimum amount recommended by doctors. But that doesn't mean the calcium quest is a wild foods chase.

Doctors and nutritionists are quick to point out that just a few foods can cause a quantum leap in your calcium level. Those supercharged foods include milk, yogurt and cheese. But there are other food sources as well.

"You can get what you need from your diet," says Creighton University's Dr. Robert Heaney. "And you don't even have to drink milk by the glass." To find out how to get over 1,500 milligrams of calcium in your daily diet, have a look at the menu on this page.

And that's just the beginning. The following are some other ways to mineralize your food without really trying.

Customize coffee with calcium. To build stronger bones the French way, start off your morning with some café au lait. Warm four ounces of low-fat (1 percent) milk on the stove or in the microwave, then add four ounces of brewed coffee. You'll get 150 milligrams of calcium, compared to the usual 37 from two tablespoons of milk.

Double the dose. Your favorite reduced-fat Alfredo sauce can benefit your bones even more. Substitute evaporated skim milk for the cream, milk or even the low-fat milk that you usually use to make the sauce.

"The advantage of using evaporated skim milk is that you more than double the amount of calcium over regular milk, not to mention cutting fat. And it gives your sauce more body than regular skim milk," says Mona Sutnick, R.D., a nutritionist in Philadelphia.

You don't have to confine Alfredo sauce to your fettuccine. Its lightly cheesy creaminess can dress up steamed cauliflower, broccoli and other vegetables. And its short list of ingredients—milk, cheese and your choice of seasonings—makes it a cinch to prepare.

A BONE-FRIENDLY MENU

At no extra charge you can charge up your daily menu with calcium-rich foods from field, farm and dairy barn. Here's a one-day menu that has all the ingredients you need for healthy bones.

Meal	Calcium (mg.)
1 cup raisin bran cereal	19
1 cup skim milk	302
2 slices cracked wheat bread, toasted	22
1 teaspoon margarine	1
1 tablespoon preserves	4
½ papaya	60
Salad with:	
¼ cup (1 oz.) cooked pinto beans	32
¼ cup (1 oz.) cooked navy beans	45
½ cup (2 oz.) steamed broccoli	26
¼ cup (1 oz.) skim mozzarella cheese	192
¼ cup (1 oz.) enriched vegetable macaroni	9
3 Tbsp. low-calorie French dressing	5
French roll	35
1 cup orange juice	103
¾ cup nonfat vanilla yogurt	300
2 oz. roasted lean pork tenderloin	5
½ cup potatoes au gratin	146
½ cup boiled turnip greens	125
Tossed green salad with:	26
¼ cup (1 oz.) grated Parmesan and Romano cheese	318
1 Tbsp. Italian dressing	1
½ cup cooked rhubarb	174
Day's Total : 1,950	

BEST AND WORST CALCIUM BETS

It's never too early, or too late, to help your bones get the calcium they need—especially if you have the right foods on your bone-building shopping list. Here are some best bets on the calcium scale—and, by contrast, some of the "worst" foods, those that provide little or none of the valuable mineral.

	Food	Portion	Calcium (mg.)	Comments
A +	*Yogurt (from skim milk)*	*8 oz.*	*414*	*Dairy products are by far the richest in calcium,*
	Skim milk	*1 cup*	*351*	*and that calcium is also easily absorbed by the*
	Buttermilk	*1 cup*	*285*	*body. Depend on them to achieve recommended*
	Mozzarella cheese (skim milk)	*1 oz.*	*180*	*calcium intake.*
A	*Sardines*	*7*	*321*	*Good supplementary calcium sources. They're high*
	Pink salmon, canned with bones	*3 oz.*	*181*	*in calcium because of the tiny bones, but sardines can also be high in fat.*
B +	*Kale, chopped, cooked*	*½ cup*	*85*	*Greens and beans are moderately high in calcium,*
	Bok choy, shredded, cooked	*½ cup*	*79*	*and that calcium is available to the body. Unfortu-*
	Mustard greens, chopped, cooked	*½ cup*	*52*	*nately, you'd have to eat mounds of them to meet*
	Broccoli, chopped, cooked	*½ cup*	*47*	*the daily calcium levels that experts recommend.*
	Pinto beans, cooked	*½ cup*	*40*	*Depend on them as supplementary calcium sources.*
	Kidney beans, cooked	*½ cup*	*25*	
	Figs, dried	*5*	*135*	*Like greens and beans, nuts and dried fruits are*
	Almonds, toasted, unblanched	*1 oz.*	*75*	*good as a supplementary source of calcium, but*
	Hazelnuts	*16 (1 oz.)*	*53*	*you'd have to cover your plate with them to meet*
	Brazil nuts	*6 (1 oz.)*	*50*	*daily requirements. Also, nuts are high in fat, and*
	Prunes, dried	*5*	*21*	*dried fruits are loaded with calories.*
F	*Spinach, cooked*	*½ cup*	*122*	*Spinach is high in oxalic acid, which makes its calcium unavailable to the body.*
	Meats			*Insignificant calcium content.*

Pump up the mashed potatoes. Beat some nonfat dry milk powder into your mashed potatoes, suggests Sutnick. Often people add about ½ cup of milk to a bowl of mashed potatoes that serves four. If you add ¼ cup of dry milk powder along with the usual amount of regular milk, you can count up an extra 208 milligrams of calcium.

Sprinkle your salad. For a quick way to add calcium to salads any time, keep a container of grated, fresh, low-fat cheese in the refrigerator. Bring the cheese bowl to the table, or sprinkle some cheese on your tossed salad just before serving.

Keep cheese chunks for crackers. If you're having cheese and crackers before dinner, cut the cheese into chunks. You'll get a good dose of calcium before you even sit down to eat.

To reach or stay above the fracture threshold, most doctors recommend that men and women get a minimum of 800 to 1,000 milligrams of calcium per day—which is approximately the equivalent of three eight-ounce glasses of skim milk. (While children can get somewhat less, it's been found that a diet high in calcium is critical to building bone reserves in children, particularly for young girls who will lose the most in their postmenopausal years.) For postmenopausal women who are not on HRT, the calcium requirement soars to 1,500 milligrams per day, the equivalent of five eight-ounce glasses of skim milk.

In addition to a calcium-rich diet, plenty of weight-bearing exercise—such as brisk walking—can also stimulate bones to maintain density. On the other hand, some of the habits we develop in our folly-filled youth can sharply increase the danger of osteoporosis. Smoking is one of them; studies show that regular smokers have 10 to 12 percent less bone density than nonsmokers. Heavy drinking is another saboteur—large doses of alcohol help erode the skeleton.

But whatever you've done—or haven't done—so far, "it's never too late for your bones," says Douglas P. Kiel, M.D., assistant professor of medicine at Harvard Medical School and director of medical research at Hebrew Rehabilitation Center for the Aged in Boston. Adding more calcium and other bone-benefiting nutrients can either help build bone or cut your losses. Just take the right tack, and you may prevent the bone fractures that many people get when they age.

MILK TO THE MAX— IN EVERY WAY

For the double benefits that good bones demand—calcium along with vitamin D—a top supplier is milk. Each eight-ounce glass of low-fat (1 percent) milk contains about 300 milligrams of calcium and 100 international units of

vitamin D—though studies have shown that the actual amount of vitamin D may differ widely from what's stated on the label.

Pairing calcium with vitamin D, doctors say, is the best dietary tactic to help halt the sneak attack of osteoporosis. Vitamin D aids in the transport of calcium across intestinal walls and into our bone cells, where it can be absorbed.

"What happens when you don't get enough vitamin D is that your bone cells happily lay down the rubbery collagen to make bone. But the collagen won't get mineralized and hard without the help of vitamin D," explains Michael F. Holick, M.D., Ph.D., director of the General Clinical Research Center at Boston University Medical Center and director of the Vitamin D Laboratory at Boston University School of Medicine.

Not only that, but "vitamin D regulates all bone density," says Nigel Morrison, Ph.D., research fellow at the Garvan Institute of Medical Research at Saint Vincent's Hospital in Sydney, Australia. "It turns on the process in the body that converts calcium to bone," he adds.

So for maximum bone-building power, milk is your best all-around bet. Here's how to get more of it.

Take it straight. If you look at the label on a carton of low-fat or skim milk, you'll see that you get about 50 percent of the vitamin D recommended by doctors in one eight-ounce glass. If that glass is low-fat (1 percent) milk, you'll get about 300 milligrams of calcium, and if it's skim you'll get 352 milligrams. With either, three or four glasses a day will put you well within range of your calcium target and give you all the vitamin D you could possibly need. (Just make sure it's low-fat or skim milk, so you don't get an overload of fat while you're boosting your calcium.)

Pack a packet. Nonfat dry milk powder has vitamin D and is packed with calcium, with 52 milligrams per tablespoon. Each packet holds about six tablespoons, so you can easily carry a day's supply in your purse, briefcase or glove compartment. Add it to tea, coffee or even some soups.

You can add as much as you want, since it contains no fat. The only trick is to first pour the hot beverage into a cup, then sprinkle on the dry powder and stir it in. If you put the powder in, then add liquid, you might get unappetizing lumps in your beverage.

Fix a fruit frappé. For a morning delight that also boosts your bone power, make a fruit frappé using evaporated skim milk.

While evaporated milk isn't very appealing on its own, blended with fruit it makes a delicious drink with 738 milligrams of calcium per cup, more than twice the amount in milk.

To make the frappé, put a cup of evaporated skim milk, a large banana and ½ cup of strawberries into a blender. For a richer taste, add ½ teaspoon of almond extract. Then whir until the ingredients are thoroughly blended.

"It's a quick, easy breakfast," says Elizabeth Ward, R.D., spokeswoman for the American Dietetic Association (ADA) and a nutritionist in Boston.

Have some backbone in your dessert. Ward has the ideal treat for people who are less than delighted with plain milk.

"I suggest they make pudding using either low-fat or skim milk and artifi-

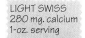

LIGHT SWISS
280 mg. calcium
1-oz. serving

LIGHT CHEDDAR
118 mg. calcium
1-oz. serving

LOW-FAT COLBY
118 mg. calcium
1-oz. serving

FETA
140 mg. calcium
1-oz. serving

LIGHT MONTEREY JACK
200 mg. calcium
1-oz. serving

PARMESAN
69 mg. calcium
1 Tbsp.

PART-SKIM MOZZARELLA
183 mg.calcium
1-oz.serving

LIGHT STRING CHEESE
200 mg. calcium
1-oz. serving

LOW-FAT, HIGH-CALCIUM CHEESES

Cheese is one of calcium's powerhouse foods, but it's usually high in fat. Usually—but not always. Some kinds are just naturally lower in fat than others, and now there are low-fat varieties that you can pick up in any supermarket.

All of the cheeses in the illustration below have less than six grams of fat per serving. But look how much calcium they contain in just a one-ounce serving, which is about a one-inch cube of cheese. (Exception: For Parmesan cheese that you usually just sprinkle on spaghetti, the calcium amount is for a tablespoon rather than an ounce.)

The next time you shop, browse through the cheese aisle and do your bones a favor by picking up some of the calcium-rich treats on this tray.

cially sweetened pudding mixes to drive the calories down," she says. In a ½-cup serving of pudding, you'll get the same vitamin D fortification and all the calcium benefits that you find in ½ cup of milk. It's a tasty low-fat dessert with bone-building power to spare.

If you're lactose intolerant, don't deny yourself milk. Some people avoid milk because of allergies that upset their digestion. But if allergies prevent you from drinking milk, you're missing a major bone builder.

Maybe you don't have to go cold turkey, advises Dr. Cooper. "Often intolerance is mild and people find they can drink up to eight ounces, spread out during the day," he observes. Try ¼ cup of milk at meals and ¼ cup in decaf or tea, he suggests. If you don't have any reactions, you may be fine at that level or even with more.

But if you're completely lactose intolerant, Dr. Cooper suggests that you try lactase, an enzyme that helps your body digest milk. Liquid lactase and chewable tablets are both available at most drugstores.

Other alternatives include lactose-reduced milk or soy-based products. They're sold at some natural food stores and supermarkets.

THE YOGURT WAY TO CALCIUM

In the calcium department, yogurt even beats milk, notes Colleen Pierre, R.D., a nutritionist in private practice in Baltimore, who is a spokeswoman for the ADA. A cup of yogurt on the average boasts about 100 more milligrams of calcium than the same amount of milk. (Yogurt's only shortcoming is that it doesn't have any of milk's vitamin D fortification.)

"Yogurt is *the* best source of calcium," agrees Paul Saltman, Ph.D., professor of biology at the University of California, San Diego.

Here are some ways high-calcium yogurt can play a part in your bone-building ensemble.

Add cereal to your yogurt. Instead of adding milk to your favorite breakfast cereal, add the cereal to low-fat yogurt. You'll gain yogurt's calcium advantage over milk. Plus, if you add cereal that's been fortified with calcium and vitamin D, you'll create a breakfast treat that will

MAKE A CHEESE TO PLEASE

Yogurt cream cheese is an easy way to get goodness to your bones. Not only is it high in calcium—with 25 to 35 milligrams per tablespoon—it's as low in fat as the yogurt it's made from. Best of all, it's easy to make. Buy any gelatin-free yogurt. (Don't use a yogurt with chunks of fruit.) To see if it will drain well, scoop out a tablespoon, then watch what happens. If liquid (whey) seeps into the depression, it should drain well enough to make cheese.

1. Line a strainer with kitchen cheesecloth, place over a medium bowl and scoop in the yogurt.

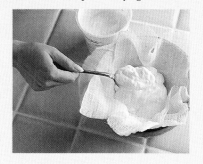

2. Cover with plastic wrap and refrigerate overnight, allowing the yogurt to drain.

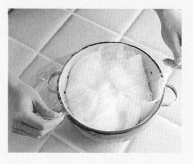

3. Then transfer the yogurt (now yogurt cheese) to a storage container and keep refrigerated.

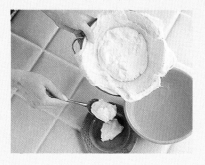

turn straight into bone benefits.

Cereal and yogurt are easier to carry to work than cereal and milk, adds Ward. So if you're used to having breakfast at the office, carry this high-calcium snack pack in your briefcase.

For a Tex-Mex bone builder, just add yogurt. South of the Border, and even north of it, many chili lovers add sour cream to their red-bean favorite. For a chili enhancer with more calcium and less fat, use yogurt instead of sour cream, suggests Jodie Shield, R.D., a spokesperson for the ADA in Chicago. The reason: Each tablespoon of yogurt has 11 milligrams more calcium than sour cream. Since the kidney beans in chili also have calcium, you're piling benefit upon benefit if you swirl a few tablespoons of yogurt into your bowl of chili.

Arrange a dip for your orange. Shield also makes a fruit dip with yogurt. Here's how: Stir two tablespoons of honey into a cup of plain nonfat yogurt, then add a dash of cinnamon and nutmeg. Peel and section an orange, then snack on orange slices dipped in the honey-yogurt mix.

Sound good? It is. And the 52 milligrams of calcium you get in an orange are rounded out by the calcium-packed yogurt you scoop with every orange section. Better yet, substitute two tablespoons of dark molasses for the honey. Molasses is an acquired taste, but you'll also acquire an additional 278 milligrams of calcium every time you use it.

WELL-CHOSEN CHEESES

Select almost any cheese, and you're tapping into a rich vein of calcium. In one ounce of cheese, you'll get about 200 milligrams of calcium, which is roughly the equivalent of two-thirds of a glass of milk. The only trouble is that when you go panning for these nuggets of calcium, you're more than likely to pick up a lot of fool's gold—fat.

But here are some tips on how to use some of the svelte new low-fat and light cheeses.

Bedeck your broccoli. "The low-fat

SIX TIPS TO GET THE MOST FROM YOUR CALCIUM SUPPLEMENT

If your calcium count usually comes up short, don't leave your bones gasping for more. Supplements are available at any pharmacy or health food store. Wondering which supplement to choose? Here are some tips from doctors.

■ *Both calcium carbonate and calcium citrate are good choices.*

■ *On the label, the words "elemental calcium" tell you how much calcium from each tablet your body can use. It's the amount that's not carbonate or citrate.*

■ *Look for a label that says "meets U.S. Pharmacopoeia (USP) standards." That's an assurance that the tablet will dissolve easily.*

■ *If USP approval is not indicated on the label, test the supplement by dropping a tablet in a glass of warm water. It should dissolve in an hour. If not, it probably won't dissolve in your body either—so you'll want to avoid buying that brand in the future.*

■ *For maximum effectiveness, take a calcium supplement with meals, recommends Dr. Michael Holick of the Boston University Medical Center.*

■ *If you're taking more than one supplement, take calcium and the other supplements in small doses at different meals to enhance absorption, suggests Dr. Robert Lindsay, president of the National Osteoporosis Foundation.*

cheeses melt well because they're processed," says Shield. That means you can make broccoli with cheese sauce in a breeze.

For each serving of broccoli, grate or shred one ounce of light cheddar cheese. Let it reach room temperature. Steam the broccoli for about five minutes, put it in a serving bowl, then scatter the grated cheese over the broccoli. Stir until the cheese melts and serve. The net gain is a whopping 118 milligrams of calcium.

Enrich Caesar. If you're a fan of Caesar salad, modify one key element and you'll be able to do your bones a favor. Next time you make a salad, try substituting one ounce of light Swiss cheese (with 280 milligrams of calcium per ounce) for the usual tablespoon of Parmesan cheese (138 milligrams per ounce).

For a topping swap, trade bacon for cheese. If you're fishing for toppings at the salad bar, skip the bacon bits and go for the bone-building cheese selections. Most salad bars offer shredded Swiss cheese, which has a lot less fat than bacon—and an ounce of it (about two tablespoons) gives you a dose of calcium that's nearly equivalent to a cup of milk.

BONING UP ON LABELS

First, cereal makers began adding calcium. Then orange juice producers got on the bone-building bandwagon. Now some brands of bread and fruit punch have joined the growing ranks of calcium-fortified foods. As calcium enters the mainstream of additional everyday foods, here's how to take advantage of the new sources.

Say okay to some OJ. Only a few brands of orange juice are calcium fortified. But wherever you find name-brand orange juices, you'll probably find at least one that's been fortified with calcium and says so, boldly, on the label. An eight-ounce glass of fortified juice contains about 300 milligrams of calcium.

Give your bones a punch lunch. A few fruit punches have been fortified with calcium. Some have over 150 milligrams of calcium per cup.

But does added calcium do the job?

A number of fortified fruit drinks and juices have been tested, and researchers concluded that calcium "gets into the bones just as well as the calcium from milk, at least judging from preliminary studies," says Dr. Rosen of the Maine Center for Osteoporosis Research.

HOW TO NET MORE

If you're fishing to find calcium in food, take a turn for the deep blue sea—and prepare to dive into some fish and shellfish. Davey Jones has a lockerful of calcium. But you have to be selective if you're going for the best of the ocean's bounty. Here's how to choose and prepare the catch.

Savor the shellfish. Clams, blue crabs, shrimp and lobster all have respectable amounts of calcium, points out Robert A. Heaney, M.D., professor

of medicine at Creighton University School of Medicine in Omaha and chairman of the U.S. Office of Technology Assessment's scientific advisory panel on osteoporosis. Blue crabs, for example, contain 88 milligrams of calcium in a three-ounce portion. (A reminder, though: Blue crabs are high in sodium, so don't go overboard eating them if you're watching your blood pressure.)

Crave the crunchies. Fish with edible bones, like sardines and canned salmon, are good sources of calcium just because you're chomping on *their* high-calcium bones every time you take a bite. But with both these fish, salt and other ingredients can be a problem. Canned sardines need to be rinsed well to flush out some of the fat and salt. And when choosing salmon, simply be sure to pick the cans that say low-salt on their labels.

Better your bones with salmon salad. Instead of a tuna fish sandwich, make one with canned salmon, which has 181 milligrams of calcium in a three-ounce portion. (Reminder: Be a lazy-bones and don't pick out the calcium-rich edible bones that will help *your* bones.)

For a delectable salmon salad, mash the salmon and add yogurt or yogurt cheese to suit your taste. You'll spice up the flavor if you add about a teaspoon of chopped fresh dill per serving. Serve it on a sandwich (between calcium-fortified white bread for an extra dose) or on a bed of dark lettuce.

THE BONE-BUILDING GARDEN

Out in the Good-Bones Garden, the broccoli is glistening, the kale is waving and the Chinese cabbage (bok choy) bares its lofty head to the sun, while collard and mustard greens rustle their dark-hued leaves. All these dark leafy greens can contribute some calcium to our diet.

But there's another good reason for choosing the dark greens. "Just about anything that's green has chlorophyll—

and the mineral in chlorophyll is magnesium," says Henry C. Lukaski, Ph.D., supervisory research physiologist at the U.S. Department of Agriculture Human Nutrition Research Center in Grand Forks, North Dakota. Magnesium is one of the minerals that's important in building bone. We usually get enough magnesium in our daily meals, and we also get significant amounts from beverages, especially water.

So before you leaf past the dark green produce in search of pale iceberg lettuce, remember these calcium and magnesium boosters.

Break out the broccoli. Broccoli has 72 milligrams of calcium per cooked cup. But you'll get even more bone-building benefits if you serve it in cream of broccoli soup. Just use your favorite recipe for the soup, but substitute half evaporated skim milk and half regular skim milk for the milk or cream that you usually use. You can hike the calcium even more by adding one tablespoon of nonfat dry milk powder to each cup of soup.

Stop at the kale counter. When people see kale in the supermarket, they notice its pretty multicolored leaves but often pass it by. The next time you see it, stop—it's got 170 milligrams of calcium per cooked cup.

Kale is one of nutritionist Colleen Pierre's favorite foods. If you are trying it for the first time, she suggests adding it to vegetable soup such as minestrone. If you're making a quart of soup, add one cup of kale 15 minutes before the soup is done.

CUTTING THE CALCIUM CUTTHROATS

While you're campaigning for more calcium in your diet, you might as well watch out for the dietary villains that can shanghai your supply—among them, alcohol and salt. These are by far the greatest calcium thieves. While you don't have to cut them completely, here are some tactics to make sure your bone bank is safe.

CAFFEINE AND CALCIUM: WAR OR TRUCE?

After a study in 1982 linked caffeine consumption with calcium loss, it looked like coffee might end up on the least-wanted list. Coffee drinkers groaned, fearing the breakfast table would turn into a caffeine-free zone. But further studies granted a reprieve.

"All the studies have shown for certain is that caffeine lowers bone density only in women who don't drink milk—who are deficient in calcium," says Michael R. McClung, M.D., director of the Osteoporosis Research Center in Portland, Oregon.

But along with having a glass of milk a day to offset the effects of caffeine, doctors say it's a good idea to moderate your coffee consumption.

"Two to three cups of coffee—or its equivalent—will probably not be of much consequence," according to researcher Dr. Douglas Kiel of Harvard Medical School. But he warns that drinking amounts in excess of that may be a problem.

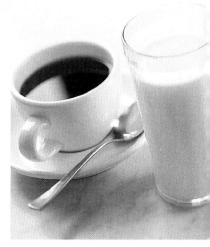

Keep a low bar bill. While an occasional drink might not hurt, you should keep in mind that alcohol hampers our bone-building ability, according to Dr. Cooper. The problem is that alcohol interferes with osteoblasts, those workaholic cells that are constantly rebuilding our bones. And when the osteoblast cells begin slacking off, our skeletons suffer the consequences.

According to Dr. Cooper, we should limit the amount of alcohol we consume to no more than ten drinks per week. (One drink means 12 ounces of beer, a 5-ounce glass of wine or a cocktail with 1½ to 2 ounces of hard liquor.)

Shake once, not twice. People who get a lot of salt in their diet may end up calcium deficient, according to Dr. Heaney. That's because salt is flushed out in the urine—and a lot of calcium is washed away with it.

If you're used to having salt on your food, try half your customary amount. Ideally, you should get no more than 1,800 milligrams of salt per day, or the equivalent of just a little less than one teaspoon. Or try one of the reduced-sodium salt substitutes. (Since salt reduction is also an important factor in lowering high blood pressure, be sure to check the tips in chapter 2.)

Credits

Photography Credits

Cover: Chris Harvey/Tony Stone Worldwide (center); Alison Miksch (top right); Angelo Caggiano (center right and bottom right)
Contents Page: *salad plate*—photographer: Alison Miksch; food and prop stylist: Kay Lichthardt
bananas—photographer: Karen Capucilli
woman with vegetables—photographer: Julia Smith
teacup—photographer: Rita Maas; food stylist: Brett Kurzweil; prop stylist: Susan Byrnes
couple at breakfast—photographer: RSI/Sally Ann Ullman
bamboo steamer—photographer: Alan Richardson; prop stylist: Denise Canter

Photographers: Allstock/Karl Weatherly: p. 98; Peter Arnold/Manfred Kage: p. 119; Peter Arnold/David Scharf: p. 96; Angelo Caggiano: pp. 3, 9 (top right), 22–23, 32–33, 36–37 (left), 38, 41 (right column), 47, 49, 54–55, 61, 111, 112, 127, 134–35, 156; Karen Capucilli: pp. 8–9, 12–13, 60, 72–73, 91, 142; Lahoma Davis: p. 140 (left); Karen Faye: p. 63; FPG/Dave Bartruff: p. 105 (left); FPG/Thomas Craig: p. 66; FPG/C. R. Rathe: p. 57; Deborah Jones: p. 78; Albert M. Kligman, M.D., Ph.D.: p. 99; Rita Maas: pp. 24, 71, 128–29, 144–45; Magnum Photos, Inc./Reno Burri: p. 105 (right); Magnum Photos, Inc./Leonard Freed: p. 53; Alison Miksch: pp. 26, 37, 84–85, 95, 106–7, 108, 114–15, 116, 124–25, 155; Ruby Nelson: p. 140 (right); Outline Press/Gerardo Somoza: p. 132; Pacific Stock/David Copwell: p. 82; Christian Peacock: p. 52; Photonica/Carol Whaley: p. 126; Photo Researchers/Dr. A. Liepins: p. 104; Alan Richardson: pp. x–1, 5, 9 (bottom right), 14, 40–41 (all but right column); RSI/John P. Hamel: p. 29 (photo manipulation by Tim Teahan), 51; RSI/Sally Ann Ullman: p. 16; David Seltzer: pp. 42–43; Chip Simons: pp. 58–59; Julia Smith: pp. 140–41; Walter Smith: pp. 86–87, 138, 149; Mark Tuschman: p. 10; Bill Westheimer: p. 7

Prop Stylists: Nathan Bodden: p. 86; Susan Byrnes: pp. 7, 24, 71, 128–29, 144–45; Denise Canter: pp. 1, 5, 9, 14, 40–41, 134–35; Francine Matalon Deigny: pp. 22–23, 26, 33, 38, 47, 49, 54–55, 95, 108, 111, 112, 114, 116, 124, 127, 155, 156; Susan Justus: p. 29; Kay Lichthardt: pp. 84–85

Food Stylists: Nathan Bodden: p. 86; Rick Ellis: pp. 22–23, 38, 41 (right), 112, 127, 134–35, 156; Brett Kurzweil: pp. 24, 95, 108, 114, 124; Kay Lichthardt: pp. 37, 84–85; Marian Sauvion: pp. 7, 8, 12, 33, 36, 49, 54–55, 91, 125; William Smith: pp. 1, 5, 9, 14, 26, 40–41, 71, 128–29, 144–45, 155

Illustration Credits

Contents Page: Narda Lebo

Linda Bleck: p. 4 and throughout ("Breakthroughs in Healing" logo); Raul Febles: p. 151 (chart); John and Linda Gist: pp. 22, 36, 37, 109; Larry Greiner: p. 32; Narda Lebo: pp. 2, 19, 30, 45, 53, 64, 68, 81, 88, 100, 107, 136, 143, 148, 150; Tim Teahan: p. 17

Index

Note: Underscored page references indicate boxed text. **Boldface** references indicate tables and charts.